New Technologies in Foot and Ankle Surgery

Editor

STEPHEN A. BRIGIDO

CLINICS IN PODIATRIC MEDICINE AND SURGERY

www.podiatric.theclinics.com

Consulting Editor
THOMAS J. CHANG

January 2018 • Volume 35 • Number 1

ELSEVIER

1600 John F. Kennedy Boulevard • Suite 1800 • Philadelphia, Pennsylvania, 19103-2899

http://www.theclinics.com

CLINICS IN PODIATRIC MEDICINE AND SURGERY Volume 35, Number 1
January 2018 ISSN 0891-8422, ISBN-13: 978-0-323-56653-7

Editor: Lauren Boyle
Developmental Editor: Meredith Madeira

Clinics in Podiatric Medicine and Surgery (ISSN 0891-8422) is published quarterly by Elsevier Inc., 360 Park Avenue South, New York, NY 10010-1710. Months of issue are January, April, July, and October. Business and Editorial Offices: 1600 John F. Kennedy Blvd., Ste. 1800, Philadelphia, PA 19103-2899. Customer Service Office: 3251 Riverport Lane, Maryland Heights, MO 63043. Periodicals postage paid at New York, NY and additional mailing offices. Subscription prices are $294.00 per year for US individuals, $544.00 per year for US institutions, $100.00 per year for US students and residents, $382.00 per year for Canadian individuals, $657.00 for Canadian institutions, $439.00 for international individuals, $657.00 per year for international institutions and $220.00 per year for Canadian and foreign students/residents. To receive student/resident rate, orders must be accompanied by name of affiliated institution, date of term, and the *signature* of program/residency coordinator on institution letterhead. Orders will be billed at individual rate until proof of status is received. Foreign air speed delivery is included in all *Clinics* subscription prices. All prices are subject to change without notice. POSTMASTER: Send address changes to *Clinics in Podiatric Medicine and Surgery*, Elsevier Health Sciences Division, Subscription Customer Service, 3251 Riverport Lane, Maryland Heights, MO 63043. **Customer Service: 1-800-654-2452 (US). From outside of the US, call 314-447-8871. Fax: 314-447-8029. E-mail: JournalsCustomerService-usa@elsevier.com (for print support); JournalsOnlineSupport-usa@elsevier.com (for online support).**

Reprints. For copies of 100 or more of articles in this publication, please contact the Commercial Reprints Department, Elsevier Inc., 360 Park Avenue South, New York, NY 10010-1710. Tel.: 212-633-3874; Fax: 212-633-3820; E-mail: reprints@elsevier.com.

Clinics in Podiatric Medicine and Surgery is covered in *MEDLINE/PubMed (Index Medicus)* and *EMBASE/Excerpta Medica*.

Contributors

CONSULTING EDITOR

THOMAS J. CHANG, DPM
Clinical Professor and Past Chairman, Department of Podiatric Surgery, California College of Podiatric Medicine, Faculty, The Podiatry Institute, Redwood Orthopedic Surgery Associates, Santa Rosa, California, USA

EDITOR

STEPHEN A. BRIGIDO, DPM, FACFAS
Section Chief, Department Chair, and Fellowship Director, Foot and Ankle Reconstruction, Department of Foot and Ankle Surgery, Coordinated Health, Bethlehem, Pennsylvania, USA; Clinical Professor of Surgery, Geisinger Commonwealth School of Medicine, Scranton, Pennsylvania, USA

AUTHORS

BOB BARAVARIAN, DPM, FACFAS
Assistant Clinical Professor, UCLA David Geffen School of Medicine, Director, University Foot & Ankle Institute, Los Angeles, California, USA

GREGORY C. BERLET, MD
Orthopedic Foot and Ankle Surgeon, Orthopedic Foot & Ankle Center, Westerville, Ohio, USA

KAITLYN BERNHARD, DPM
Third Year Resident, PMSR/RRA, Highlands/Presbyterian St. Luke's Podiatric Surgical Residency Program, Denver, Colorado, USA

ROBERTO A. BRANDÃO, DPM
Foot and Ankle Fellow, Orthopedic Foot & Ankle Center, Westerville, Ohio, USA

STEPHEN A. BRIGIDO, DPM, FACFAS
Section Chief, Department Chair, and Fellowship Director, Foot and Ankle Reconstruction, Department of Foot and Ankle Surgery, Coordinated Health, Bethlehem, Pennsylvania, USA; Clinical Professor of Surgery, Gelsinger Commonwealth School of Medicine, Scranton, Pennsylvania, USA

PATRICK E. BULL, DO
Orthopedic Foot and Ankle Surgeon, Orthopedic Foot & Ankle Center, Westerville, Ohio, USA

SCOTT C. CARRINGTON, DPM
Fellow, Foot and Ankle Reconstruction, Department of Foot and Ankle Surgery, Coordinated Health, Bethlehem, Pennsylvania, USA

THOMAS J. CHANG, DPM
Clinical Professor and Past Chairman, Department of Podiatric Surgery, California College of Podiatric Medicine, Faculty, The Podiatry Institute, Redwood Orthopedic Surgery Associates, Santa Rosa, California, USA

JAMES M. COTTOM, DPM, FACFAS
Director, Florida Orthopedic Foot & Ankle Center Fellowship, Florida Orthopedic Foot & Ankle Center, Sarasota, Florida, USA

PAUL DAYTON, DPM, MS, FACFAS
Assistant Professor, Department of Podiatric Medicine and Surgery, College of Podiatric Medicine and Surgery, Des Moines University, UnityPoint Health, Trinity Regional Medical Center, Des Moines, Iowa, USA

LAWRENCE DiDOMENICO, DPM, FACFAS
Director, Reconstructive Rearfoot and Ankle Surgical Fellowship, Director of Residency Training, Northside Regional Medical Center, Section Chief, St. Elizabeth's Medical Center, Youngstown, Ohio, USA

ZACHARY FLYNN, DPM, AACFAS
Fellow, Reconstructive Rearfoot and Ankle Surgical Fellowship, St. Elizabeth's Medical Center, Youngstown, Ohio, USA

DANIEL J. HATCH, DPM, FACFAS
Director of Surgical Training, Department of Podiatric Medicine and Surgery, North Colorado PMS Residency, Greeley, Colorado, USA

CHRISTOPHER F. HYER, DPM, MS, FACFAS
Fellowship Director of the Orthopedic Foot and Ankle Center Fellowship, Fellowship Trained Foot and Ankle Surgeon, Orthopedic Foot & Ankle Center, Westerville, Ohio, USA

GUIDO A. LaPORTA, DPM, MS, FACFAS
Department of Graduate Medical Education and Podiatric Surgery, Our Lady of Lourdes Memorial Hospital, Binghamton, New York, USA

DAVID LARSON, DPM, AACFAS
Fellowship Trained Foot and Ankle Surgeon, Integrated Orthopedics, Phoenix, Arizona, USA

TAL PNINA LINDNER, PhD
Vice President, Scientific and Regulatory Affairs, Ossio Ltd, Tel Aviv, Israel

JEFFREY E. McALISTER, DPM, FACFAS
Attending Physician, The CORE Institute, Phoenix, Arizona, USA

BRYON McKENNA, DPM
Department of Surgery, Mount Auburn Hospital, Cambridge, Massachusetts, USA; Clinical Fellow of Surgery, Harvard Medical School, Boston, Massachusetts, USA

RONIT MERCHAV-FEUERMANN, DVM
Medical Director, Ossio Ltd, Tel Aviv, Israel

ALAN NG, DPM, FACFAS
Attending Physician, PMSR/RRA, Highlands/Presbyterian St. Luke's Podiatric Surgical Residency Program, Private Practice, Advanced Orthopedic and Sports Medicine Specialists, Denver, Colorado, USA

DAVID I. PEDOWITZ, MS, MD
Associate Professor, Department of Orthopaedic Surgery, Thomas Jefferson Medical College, The Rothman Institute, Philadelphia, Pennsylvania, USA

MURRAY J. PENNER, MD, FRCS(C)
Professor, Orthopedic Foot and Ankle Surgeon, Department of Orthopedic Surgery, The University of British Columbia, Vancouver, British Columbia, Canada

BRITTON S. PLEMMONS, DPM, AACFAS
Fellow, Florida Orthopedic Foot & Ankle Center, Sarasota, Florida, USA

MARK A. PRISSEL, DPM, AACFAS
Fellowship Trained Foot and Ankle Surgeon, Orthopedic Foot & Ankle Center, Westerville, Ohio, USA

NICOLE M. PROTZMAN, MS
Research Associate, Clinical Integration Department, Coordinated Health, Allentown, Pennsylvania, USA

MICHAEL REED, DPM
Resident, Northside Regional Medical Center, Youngstown, Ohio, USA

RYAN B. RIGBY, DPM, FACFAS
Attending Physician, Logan Regional Orthopedics, Logan, Utah, USA

ROBERT D. SANTROCK, MD
Assistant Professor and Chief of Foot and Ankle Surgery, Department of Orthopaedics, West Virginia University, Morgantown, West Virginia, USA

RYAN T. SCOTT, DPM, FACFAS
Attending Physician, The CORE Institute, Phoenix, Arizona, USA

W. BRET SMITH, DO, MS
Director of Foot and Ankle Division, Palmetto Health USC Orthopedic Center, Assistant Professor, Orthopedics, University of South Carolina, Lexington, South Carolina, USA

N. JAKE SUMMERS, DPM
Dartmouth-Hitchcock, Foot and Ankle/Podiatry, Bedford, New Hampshire, USA

JUSTIN TSAI, MS, MD
Assistant Professor, Department of Orthopaedic Surgery, SUNY Downstate College of Medicine, Brooklyn, New York, USA

FERAS J. WALY, MBBS, FRCS(C)
Orthopedic Foot and Ankle Fellow, Department of Orthopaedic Surgery, St Paul's Hospital, Vancouver, British Columbia, Canada; Orthopedic Surgeon, Department of Orthopedic Surgery, University of Tabuk, Tabuk, Saudi Arabia

JEFFREY S. WEBER, DPM, AACFAS
Fellowship Trained Foot and Ankle Surgeon, Milwaukee Foot and Ankle Specialists, New Berlin, Wisconsin, USA

JESSICA L. WILCZEK, DPM
Department of Graduate Medical Education and Podiatric Surgery, Our Lady of Lourdes Memorial Hospital, Binghamton, New York, USA

NICHOLAS E. YEO, MBBS, FRCS
Orthopedic Foot and Ankle Fellow, Department of Orthopaedic Surgery, St Paul's Hospital, Vancouver, British Columbia, Canada; Associate Consultant, Department of Orthopaedic Surgery, Singapore General Hospital, Singapore, Singapore

Contents

> Amnion and amniotic tissue has been studied for more than 100 years in the treatment of acute and chronic wounds. Recent studies have focused on the use of amnion tissue in the management of full-thickness diabetic wounds, particularly of the lower extremities. With new harvesting, processing, and distribution technologies, amnion is increasingly available in treating these wounds. Current data and research show increased healing potential and decreased healing times, pain, drainage, and infection in wounds treated with amnion products. There are a variety of amnion products with varying differences and purposes, requiring additional research and comparison trials.

> Particulated juvenile allograft cartilage (PJAC) has significant promise and is currently supported by several studies. Potential benefits of this new technique include single-stage procedure, simplicity in the surgical technique, implantation of juvenile tissue, and a lack of donor site morbidity. This article discusses the imaging, surgical options, and postoperative management of PJAC.

> Bone marrow aspirate has been used for the adjunctive treatment of numerous pathologic conditions in orthopedics. Viable cells are found in aspiration from many different anatomic regions of the body. Concentration of these cells has been shown to improve healing due to the increased number of certain important cells. This article discusses the mechanisms involved and reviews the literature.

> Hallux-abducto-valgus or "bunion" surgery is one of the most common surgical procedures for the foot and ankle specialist. As our understanding

of the hallux-abducto-valgus deformity has grown, it is becoming clear that the anatomic CORA of the deformity may lie at the tarsometatarsal joint. There is also the component of the 3-dimensional nature of the deformity that may be best addressed at this CORA. With these issues in mind, it was necessary to address the shortcomings of the traditional Lapidus procedure and progress toward more consistent, instrumented steps that could address the 3-dimensional nature of the deformity.

Arthrodesis of the ankle or foot is a common procedure for chronic pain and disability. Nonunion remains a prevalent complication among arthrodesis procedures. Some patients present with an inherent risk of developing a nonunion. Allograft biologics have gained popularity in an effort to reduce complications such as nonunion. Various biologics bring unique properties while maintaining a singular purpose. Platelet-derived growth factor (PDGF) may be introduced into a fusion site to facilitate healthy bony consolidation. The purpose of this article was to review the benefits and modalities of PDGF and how it can improve patient outcomes in ankle and hindfoot fusions.

Advancement in orthopedics has been increasing rapidly. The most important advances have been in fixation. With time, metallic hardware will begin to be replaced by materials that become one with the body. This progress will not only aid in the repair process, it will allow permanent and improved reinforcement of the fixated region. Biointegrative technology is a promising new generation of materials capable of achieving this goal. Over time, it is expected that plates, screws, pins, interference screws, and even possibly joint replacements will incorporate into patients' bodies, negating the need for hardware removal and adding structure and stability to an iatrogenically weakened area.

Surgical correction of complex foot and ankle deformities secondary to Charcot neuroarthropathy remains a significant surgical challenge. New technological advancements in hardware have allowed for the use of augmented fixation techniques in midfoot deformity correction, including the use of indication-specific locking plates and beaming techniques that offer enhanced stability. Severe hindfoot deformity management can use internal fixation, including intramedullary hindfoot nails and circular external fixation frames for limb salvage.

Total ankle arthroplasty is an increasingly popular procedure to address tibiotalar joint arthritis. Implant design and the rationale behind it have changed throughout the years. Newer generation implants allow for minimal resection of bone and use fixed-bearing technology. Long-term follow-up multicenter studies will determine the lifetime of these devices and their effectiveness in addressing pain and improving function for patients with endstage tibiotalar arthritis.

Total ankle replacement (TAR) has evolved over the past decade as a treatment for end-stage ankle arthritis with improved survivorship. Despite the improving outcomes, ankle deformity represents a challenge to the foot and ankle surgeon with increased risk of implant failure. The use of preoperative computer-assisted guidance has led to better understanding the 3-dimensional ankle anatomy and associated deformities and allows for reproducible, anatomic placement of the TAR components.

Prolonged or incomplete healing of the foot and ankle can pose significant challenges. Therefore, investigators have begun searching for alternative treatment strategies. With advances in tissue engineering, decellularized human placental connective tissue matrix has been suggested as a means to achieve more rapid and complete healing for various soft tissue and bone procedures. Basic science and clinical studies have shown that decellularized human placental connective tissue matrix can support regenerative healing through cellular migration, accelerated tissue remodeling, and the establishment of functional tissue. Additional research is needed to fully explore and evaluate clinical applications within the foot and ankle.

Charcot deformity is a challenge that foot and ankle surgeons struggle to manage successfully. Despite the advances in knowledge, technology, and treatment modalities, limb loss is still greater than 10%. This article discusses the efficacy of conservative measures and traditional surgical approaches. It proposes a multidisciplinary team approach, medical optimization, and lifestyle modification to put the patient in the best position to heal. Also discussed is the authors' staged surgical treatment protocol to enhance outcomes and decrease the rate of limb loss.

Limb deformity correction has been widely discussed in orthopedic litera-ture with an increasing interest in technologically based surgical strate-gies. However, principles described by Ilizarov and Paley still form the basis of these newly developing surgical systems. The recent advances and increased use of computers and mobile devices in the medical arena, along with the application of dynamic hexapod external fixation, have allowed for easier and more convenient strategies, leading to a greater outreach and more confidence in the newer surgeon when faced with addressing a patient with a limb deformity.

The Cartiva implant is an exciting option in dramatically diminishing patient symptoms in advanced stages of hallux rigidus as well as allowing continued joint motion. The procedure does not burn many bridges in case a future revision to an arthrodesis is necessary. This advantage is in contradistinction to other current implants whereby more bone resection is required for implant placement.

CLINICS IN PODIATRIC MEDICINE AND SURGERY

RELATED INTEREST

Foot and Ankle Clinics, March 2017 (Vol. 22, Issue 1)
Current Controversies in Foot and Ankle Trauma
Michael P. Swords, *Editor*
Available at: http://www.foot.theclinics.com/

THE CLINICS ARE AVAILABLE ONLINE!
Access your subscription at:
www.theclinics.com

Foreword

New Technologies in Foot and Ankle Surgery

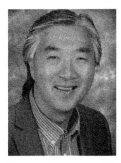

Thomas J. Chang, DPM
Consulting Editor

It is with great honor that I assume the position of Consulting Editor for the *Clinics of Podiatric Medicine and Surgery*. My sincere congratulations go out to Dr Thomas Zgonis for an outstanding job over the past years in this role. Throughout my career, I have often read and consulted with this publication on cutting-edge and review articles on a variety of topics that piqued my interest. I hope we can now pique your interest and stimulate further education. I am excited to work alongside the editorial board in the upcoming years to bring new and exciting topics to the readers, and I welcome your feedback and communication.

This first issue is called "New Technologies in Foot and Ankle Surgery." I was especially pleased Dr Steven Brigido accepted the role of Guest Editor for this issue. He is extremely involved in cutting-edge research and has a keen sense of the new technologies, which drive the foot and ankle space. He has compiled an exceptional list of topics and authors who have shared their own excitement in their specialty areas. I applaud the efforts of Dr Brigido and his list of authors in sharing their expertise with the readers.

New technologies will continue to stimulate our knowledge base and cause us to reevaluate our current approaches. Not every new technology will truly offer any new benefits from their older counterparts. We owe it to ourselves and our patients to evaluate each carefully, with an objective look at potential positives and negatives. Efficiency and practicality of utilization, cost of the new products, and ultimately,

Clin Podiatr Med Surg 35 (2018) xiii–xiv
https://doi.org/10.1016/j.cpm.2017.09.001
0891-8422/18/© 2017 Published by Elsevier Inc.

patient outcomes are just some parameters to guide us. New technologies still require well-designed research to stand the test of time.

Enjoy this first issue of 2018.

Thomas J. Chang, DPM
Department of Podiatric Surgery
California College of Podiatric Medicine
The Podiatry Institute
Redwood Orthopedic Surgery Associates
208 Concourse Boulevard
Santa Rosa, CA 95403, USA

E-mail address:
thomaschang14@comcast.net

Preface

New Technologies in Foot and Ankle Reconstruction

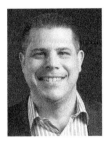

Stephen A. Brigido, DPM, FACFAS
Editor

Surgery of the foot and ankle can be one of the most complicated of the skeletal system. With many small bones and joints, surgical reconstruction of disease and injury can be challenging. Over the last ten to fifteen years, the evolution of technology in foot and ankle surgery has become one of the fastest growing, if not the fastest growing, segment in orthopedic device development. Not long ago, foot and ankle surgeons were forced to adapt to use products that were developed for large joints or long bones. Conditions such as Charcot arthropathy had limited fixation tools, and complicated cases were often abandoned for amputation because of limited access to appropriate fixation. Options for patients that were suffering from degenerative joint disease of the ankle had limited options for treatment, and those patients with focal cartilage defects had almost no options for treatment.

Fast forward to 2017, and the evolution of foot and ankle fixation has changed dramatically. Technology is being developed for procedure-specific applications. Challenges that a foot and ankle surgeon once thought difficult have evolved into procedures that are now routine and take less than half the time to complete. Advancements in tissue engineering and science have allowed surgeons to supplement poor bone and tissue with new and allow for regeneration. Ankle replacement has become commonplace in foot and ankle surgery, with implants that have a longer lifespan. In the near future, foot and ankle surgeons will be able to treat bone injuries with absorbable fixation that has the rigidity and strength of metal.

I hope you find this issue of *Clinics in Podiatric Medicine and Surgery* both informative and enjoyable. The extremely talented authors discuss new advancements in foot and ankle surgery. These technologies range from new ways to treat the Charcot foot

Clin Podiatr Med Surg 35 (2018) xv–xvi
http://dx.doi.org/10.1016/j.cpm.2017.08.011
0891-8422/18/© 2017 Published by Elsevier Inc.

podiatric.theclinics.com

and the next-generation ankle replacement to advances in tissue engineering and healing.

Stephen A. Brigido, DPM, FACFAS
Department of Foot and Ankle Surgery
Coordinated Health
2775 Schoenersville Road
Bethlehem, PA 18015, USA

Geisinger Commonwealth School of Medicine
529 Pine Street
Scranton, PA 18509, USA

E-mail address:
drsbrigido@mac.com

Amnion

The Ideal Scaffold for Treating Full-Thickness Wounds of the Lower Extremity

Bryon McKenna, DPM[a], N. Jake Summers, DPM[b],*

KEYWORDS

- Amnion • Amniotic membrane • Full-thickness • Scaffold • Wounds

KEY POINTS

- Amnion-chorion tissue is an ideal scaffold for lower extremity wounds given the growth factors and protein matrix that are present.
- Use of these products is not a new concept, it was first published in the early twentieth century; however, there have been significant improvements in the safety and packaging of the tissue.
- Research has shown that using amnion in nonhealing wounds significantly improves the rate of healing and chance of complete healing.
- More research is needed comparing the different types of tissue or products.

INTRODUCTION

Amniotic tissue has been in use for chronic wounds, skin transplants, and burns since the early twentieth century when Drs Sabella,[1] Davis,[2] and Stern[3] first published on transplanting fresh amniotic tissue immediately following birth to chronic wounds and burns with pronounced response. Drs Stern and Sabella worked together performing their research; however, they published their data separately. They both harvested tissue immediately following a birth, harvesting amniotic tissue from the umbilical cord directly adjacent to the fetal tissue. They began applying the harvested amniotic tissue to wounds to aid in healing and both advocated for a wax dressing to keep the tissue in place on the wound after application. Early studies showed improved wound healing, reduced pain,[4–6] reduced fluid loss,[7,8] and reduced infection rates.[9,10] Initial utilization was performed in acute and burn wounds; however, in the late twentieth century, amniotic tissue was shown to be beneficial for treating chronic,

Disclosures: B. McKenna has nothing to disclose. N.J. Summers is a consultant and lecturer for Alliqua Biomedical.
[a] Department of Surgery, Mount Auburn Hospital, 330 Mount Auburn Street, Cambridge, MA 02138, USA; [b] Dartmouth-Hitchcock, Foot and Ankle/Podiatry, 25 South River Road, Bedford, NH 03110, USA
* Corresponding author.
E-mail address: n.jake.summers@hitchcock.org

nonhealing wounds.[11,12] The utilization and application of amniotic tissue to wounds is not a new concept; however, the availability and new applications of the products have significantly improved in recent years. The advancements are a result of new processing procedures that have allowed companies the ability to preserve the products, allowing greater availability to physicians and their patients, as well as new research evaluating the use of amniotic tissue for new purposes.

BIOCHEMICAL PROPERTIES

Harvested fetal tissue is divided in to 2 components: chorionic tissue (outer layer) and amniotic tissue (inner layer). The amniotic layer is the focus of this article and has been the primary focus of most research in this area. The amniotic layer is unique in that it does not contain any blood vessels, muscle fibers, lymphatic tissues, or nerves. The function of the amniotic tissue in fetal development is to regulate the amniotic fluid and the rest of the fetal environment.[13] The amnion is divided into 5 unique layers: epithelium, basement membrane, compact layer, fibroblast layer, and spongy (intermediate) layer.[14] The basement membrane is composed of collagens III and IV and glycoproteins, including laminin, nidogen, and fibronectin, and is noted to be a thin layer immediately deep to the epithelium.[15] The compact layer forms the main fibrous support of the amnion, composed of collagens I and III, forming bundles, and collagens V and VI, forming filamentous connections to the basement membrane.[15] The thickest layer is the fibroblast layer and is composed of nonfibrillar meshwork of collagen III and proteoglycans and glycoproteins[14] (**Table 1**).

In the 1980s and 1990s, surgeons observed that fetuses that had undergone surgical procedures were born without scar formation or inflammation.[16] This discovery led to an influx of research about amniotic tissue and the potential use for wounds and other injuries. Research has shown that amnion has an increased concentration of certain factors that propagate wound healing without scar formation and limit inflammation without inhibiting it completely. It is important to realize that the inflammatory phase of healing is a critical step; however, preventing chronic inflammation or overactivity of the inflammatory cascade is critical for wound healing. Hao and colleagues[17] evaluated the concentration of certain cytokines in amnion tissue,

Table 1
The contents of each layer of the 5 unique layers of the amnion before processing

Amnion Layer	Components
Epithelium	Epithelium
Basement membrane	Collagen III and IV Glycoproteins laminin, nidogen, and fibronectin
Compact layer	Collagen I and III Collagen V and VI
Fibroblast layer	Collagen III Proteoglycans Glycoproteins
Spongy (intermediate) layer	

Each layer plays a unique role important to the purpose of the amnion in the fetal development. The chorion is connected to the amnion at the spongy (intermediate) layer and is significantly thicker than the amnion.

Data from John T. Human amniotic membrane transplantation: past, present and future. Ophthalmol Clin North Am 2003;16:43–65; and Niknejad H, Peirovi H, Jorjani M, et al. Properties of the amniotic membrane for potential use in tissue engineering. Eur Cell Mater 2008;15:88–99.

discovering elevated amounts of interleukin (IL)-10 and IL-1 receptor antagonist (IL-1RA). IL-10 is known to promote B-cell survival, proliferation, and antibody production. IL-1RA limits the effect of IL-1, tissue inhibitor of metalloproteinases, and other key factors in the proinflammatory cascade.

Koob and colleagues[18] used enzyme-linked immunosorbent assay (ELISA) to evaluate and attempt to quantify the growth factors that are present in dehydrated human amnion-chorion membrane (dHACM) products. The study revealed quantifiable levels of the following factors:

- Platelet-derived growth factor (PDGF)-AA and PDGF-BB
- Transforming growth factor (TGF)-alpha and TGF-beta1
- Basic fibroblast growth factor
- Epidermal growth factor
- Granulocyte colony-stimulating factor.

To understand the importance of these and other factors in chronic wounds, the concept of dynamic reciprocity in cell signaling must be explored. Essentially, human tissue is broken down into 3 fundamental components: extracellular matrix; protein growth factors, including cytokines and chemokines that are bound to the extracellular matrix; and living cells. During a state of injury, the change in the levels or condition of any of these 3 components leads to reciprocal signaling between the components. During the injured state, the other 2 components restore the third component back to its normal state, resulting in normal tissue repair. External mechanical forces, such as tension or load are often considered a fourth component in this model, particularly in the lower extremities. The interaction between these cellular components resulting in normal wound healing is referred to as dynamic reciprocity.[19] The previously mentioned growth factors, including their cytokines and chemokines, present in the amniotic tissue have been shown to induce dermal fibroblast proliferation while regulating the inflammatory stage.

A study by Koob and colleagues[20] showed that amnion-chorion products express higher levels of growth factors compared with single-layer amnion products. There are no current side-by-side studies that directly compare the healing rate or efficacy of each type of product against the others, so the significance of this is unknown. Dehydrated dHACMs have been shown to express 2 stem cell recruitment and homing factors. These factors include stromal-cell derived factor 1 and chemokine receptor type 4. These properties allow the dHACM to promote the migration of mesenchymal stem cells to the wound area. This has been observed in studies evaluating the wound environment in the presence of these products.[21] These products have also been clearly found to promote angiogenesis with the presence of multiple proangiogenic factors.[22]

TYPES OF PRODUCTS

There is a wide variety of amniotic products available for treating wounds of the lower extremity, each with variations in amnion harvesting, processing, packaging, and uses. The tissue is typically harvested after a healthy, elective Caesarian section, with full informed consent by the mother before delivery. After collection of the tissue, the tissue itself goes through vigorous testing and sterilization processing before application. This is a significant improvement from when amnion tissue was first used for wound care and applied fresh after birth without testing or sterilization processing. Obviously, the risks for transmission of disease and donor site reactions were significantly higher before the new standards.

Amniotic tissue is regulated under US Food and Drug Administration (FDA) section 361, Human Cell Tissue or Products (HCT/P), under Code of Federal Regulations 21, part 1271 of the Public Health Services Act regulatory pathway. Under the FDA 361 HCT/P regulatory pathway, the tissue must be minimally manipulated and intended for homologous use, and premarket approval or clearance is not required; however, FDA Good Tissue Practices is required. Tissue donation is regulated by the American Academy of Tissue Banks for testing and screening for infectious diseases. The diseases that are required to be tested for include human immunodeficiency virus (HIV) 1 and 2 antibodies, HIV type 1 (nucleic acid test), human T-cell lymphotropic virus type 1 and 2 antibodies, hepatitis B core antibody and surface antigen, hepatitis C antibody and virus (nucleic acid test), cytomegalovirus total antibody, and syphilis (serologic test).

The available products are similar in many ways, all sharing the basic source of amnion tissue, some with combined amnion-chorion tissue. The difference in the available products begins with the processing of the tissue to allow for distribution, allowing for longer storage, more versatility for application, and strength of the material. First, products are divided based on viability of the tissue. Some are viable placental tissue, devitalized placental tissue, and decellularized placental tissue (**Fig. 1**). There are no current studies that compare the different types of amniotic tissue products against each other. As previously mentioned, it has been shown that approximately 75% of growth factors come from the much thicker chorion layer[20]; however, the clinical significance of this is difficult to assess given the lack of head-to-head comparisons between products and the similar healed rates currently reported in literature.

Next, the products available are divided based on the sterilization process that is used. The methods that are available for processing include cryopreservation, dehydration, glycerol preservation, lyophilization and gamma irradiation, ethanol sterilization and silver impregnation. The 2 most popular processes are cryopreservation and dehydration. A comparison study between fresh amnion-chorion and cryopreserved amniotic tissue was performed that found that the cryopreserved tissue had less overall total protein and serum albumin but retained the high-molecular-weight hyaluronic acid.[23] There are no current comparative studies between cryopreserved

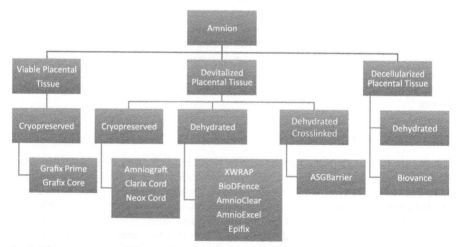

Fig. 1. There are many different types of amniotic tissue products available for use for foot and ankle wounds. The products are categorized based on the type of tissue and preservation techniques.

tissue and dehydrated tissue. Koob and colleagues[21] performed a similar study comparing the growth factor content and tissue strength before and after the dehydration process. The results showed that the tissue retained the tensile strength and the ability to promote dermal fibroblast proliferation after dehydration.

Acellular products rid the tissue of all viable cells while retaining the scaffold of the amnion and matrix of human proteins to support cellular ingrowth, whereas cellular products retain some degree of the fetal cells. The advantage of using acellular products is that it significantly decreases the risk of an immunogenic-mediated inflammatory response, as well as greater versatility for irregular wound beds. The use of acellular products is perhaps appropriate for the healthier individual who can mount an appropriate response with endogenous cells and use it as a true scaffold to promote the healing process, using and recruiting growth factors and cytokines at a biologically appropriate level. Cellular products may be more appropriate for patients with significant systemic diseases or immunocompromised individuals who may not be able to mount an appropriate response with endogenous cells. Both product types have significantly improved healing compared with standard wound care (SWC) in case studies and randomized controlled trials; however, there is no comparative study between the 2 types of products, so it is not possible to conclude that either is superior to the other, although each may have its individual pros and cons.

CLINICAL RESEARCH

There has been a significant increase in the clinical research of amniotic tissue and its application to wounds of the lower extremity. A substantial amount of early research of amniotic tissue use in wounds was performed in the ophthalmology arena, as well as in treating burns; however, the focus on lower extremities has allowed for improvement in products unique to the wound environment and strain of the extremity. Most of the research in foot and ankle applications for amniotic tissues has been performed in more recent years. Early research continues to grow but initially has consisted of small trials with small populations. One of the earliest studies is a case series published by Letendre and colleagues.[24] This was an open-label study of 14 subjects with chronic, nonhealing partial-thickness or full-thickness wounds of the lower extremities. The subjects were divided into 2 groups (partial-thickness and full-thickness wounds) and a dehydrated amnion product was applied to all wounds. The results showed 60.1%, 6 of the 9 participants who completed the entire 12-week follow-up, received benefit from use of the product, defined as decreased time to wound healing or improvement of the wounds.

Zelen and colleagues[25] conducted a single-center, randomized controlled trial that compared the use of a dHACM to SWC with an endpoint of 6 weeks. Subjects included in the study were diagnosed with a diabetic foot ulcer of at least 4 weeks duration without infection and appropriate vascular supply and were randomly split into 2 groups: dHACM (number [N] = 13) and SWC (N = 12). SWC used in the study consisted of wound debridement, appropriate moist wound therapy with the use of Silvasorb gel and Aquacel AG as needed, and a compression dressing. After 4 weeks, the wounds reduced in size by an average of 32.0% plus or minus 47.3% for SWC compared with 97.1% plus or minus 7.0% ($P<.001$) for the dHACM group. At 4 weeks and 6 weeks, the overall healed rates were 0% and 8% for SWC and 77% and 92% for dHACM groups, respectively.

Lavery and colleagues[26] performed a multicenter randomized controlled trial, including 97 participants, comparing the utilization of a cryopreserved viable placental tissue product compared with SWC. The primary endpoint of the study was complete wound healing at 12 weeks. All participants who were included were diagnosed with diabetic foot ulcers, the participants were randomized into 2 groups: SWC (N = 47) and human viable wound matrix (hVWM) (N = 50). At 12 weeks, the hVWM group had a significantly higher healed rate (60%) than the SWC group (21%, P = .0001). The median time to healing was 42 days for the hVWM group compared with 69.5 days for the SWC group. Comparing the 2 study groups, there was not a significant difference in wounds that stayed healed.

In a more recent randomized controlled study by DiDomenico and colleagues,[27] 40 subjects diagnosed with a diabetic foot ulcer were randomized into 2 groups: dHACM (N = 20) and SWC (N = 20). The primary endpoint for this study was complete wound healing at 6 weeks. At 6 weeks 70% (14/20) of the dHACM group had healed completely compared with 15% (3/20) in the SWC group. Results at 12 weeks revealed 85% (17/20) and 25% (5/20) healed in the dHACM group and SWC group, respectively. The conclusion was made that the dHACM significantly improved complete healing rates for diabetic foot ulcers, as well as increased the rate of healing as measured by time to closure.

In 2015, Smiell and colleagues[28] performed a real-world multicenter observational study in an effort to evaluate the generalizability and real-world applications of decellularized dehydrated human amniotic membrane (DDHAM) in chronic nonhealing wounds. They included all comers in their study, regardless of comorbidities, with the only exclusion being those with a known hypersensitivity to DDHAM. Because most randomized controlled trials eliminate nearly 50% of the wound populations due to inclusion or exclusion criteria, the aim was to observe the effects of DDHAM in a real-world population (N = 179) with 98% (162/166) of the chronic wounds located in the lower extremity. Their study showed more than 48% of wounds healed within a median of 6.3 weeks, including wounds that had failed previous advanced biologic therapy. Those not healed within 10.3 weeks showed a reduction in wound area of 50%. They also showed that some of the most significant factors inhibiting wound closure were the presence of infection and lack of compliance with offloading (**Table 2**).

Table 2
Evidence from recent publications evaluating amniotic tissue for nonhealing wounds of the foot and ankle

Author	Product	Study Design (Number of Subjects)	Results Healed Rate
DiDomenico et al,[27] 2016	AmnioBand	RCT (N = 40)	AmnioBand 70%, SWC 15%; 6 wk
Zelen et al,[29] 2016	Epifix, Apligraft	RCT (N = 100)	Epifix 97%, Apligraft 73%, SWC 51%
Smiell et al,[28] 2015	Biovance	Observational (N = 179)	48.8%; 6.3 wk
Serena et al,[30] 2014	Epifix	Case series (N = 20)	90% 12 wk
Lavery et al,[26] 2014	Grafix	RCT (N = 97)	Grafix 62%, SWC 21%; 12 wk
Zelen,[31] 2013	Epifix	Case series (N = 11)	91% 12 wk
Zelen et al,[25] 2013	Epifix	RCT (N = 25)	Epfix 92%, SWC 8%, 6 wk
Werber & Martin,[32] 2013	AmnioMatrix	Case series (N = 20)	90% healed 12 wk
Letendre et al,[24] 2009	Biovance	Case Series (N = 14)	60.1% benefited

Abbreviation: RCT, randomized controlled trial.

SUMMARY

Nonhealing wounds of the lower extremity are a significant problem in medicine today. The significant advancement in wound care products and, particularly, amniotic tissue has improved the treatment of the nonhealing wounds of the lower extremities considerably in recent years. There are many different types of amnion products that are available on the market for use on full-thickness ulcers of the lower extremities. Using the concept of dynamic reciprocity in wound healing, it is easier to conceptualize how amnion tissue is an ideal scaffold for these wounds. The amnion tissue facilitates an environment that replenishes and/or helps to signal and promote migration of cellular components that are needed for complete wound healing while limiting the overactivation of the inflammatory response. The use of this tissue allows for reduced scar formation, anti-inflammatory properties, introduction of matrix components, and regeneration potential with immune privilege because this tissue is not recognized as foreign. These properties allow amnion tissue to act as an ideal scaffold for lower extremity wounds. The current research has shown significant improvement in wound healing using human amnion-chorion tissue compared with SWC. Utilization of amnion allows for a faster rate of wound healing, as well as a higher percentage of complete healing. It is clear that more research is needed, particularly head-to-head comparisons between different types of tissue available; however, it is clear this should pique interest in the potential benefits human amnion-chorion tissue can provide in the healing of lower extremity full-thickness wounds.

REFERENCES

1. Sabella N. Use of fetal membranes in skin grafting. Med Records NY 1913;83: 478–80.
2. Davis JW. Skin transplantation with a review of 550 cases at the Johns Hopkins Hospital. Johns Hopkins Med J 1910;15:307–96.
3. Stern M. The grafting of preserved amniotic membrane to burned and ulcerated surfaces, substituting skin grafts. JAMA 1913;60:973–8.
4. Gajiwala K, Gajiwala AL. Evaluation of lyophilized, gamma-irradiated amnion as a biological dressing. Cell Tissue Bank 2004;5(2):73–80.
5. Gajiwala K, Lobo Gajiwala A. Use of banked tissue in plastic surgery. Cell Tissue Bank 2003;4(2–4):141–6.
6. Mermet I, Pottier N, Sainthillier JM, et al. Use of amniotic membrane transplantation in the treatment of venous leg ulcers. Wound Repair Regen 2007;15(4): 459–64.
7. Herndon DN, Thompson PB, Desai MH, et al. Treatment of burns in children. Pediatr Clin North Am 1985;32(5):1311–32.
8. May SR. The effects of biological wound dressings on the healing process. Clin Mater 1991;8(3–4):243–9.
9. Bose B. Burn wound dressing with human amniotic membrane. Ann R Coll Surg Engl 1979;61(6):444–7.
10. Ravishanker R, Bath AS, Roy R. "Amnion Bank" – the use of long term glycerol preserved amniotic membranes in the management of superficial and superficial partial thickness burns. Burns 2003;29(4):369–74.
11. Pesteil F, Oujaou-Faiz K, Drouet M, et al. Cryopreserved amniotic membrane use in resistant vascular ulcers. J Mal Vasc 2007;32(4–5):201–9.

12. Singh R, Chouhan US, Purohit S, et al. Radiation processed amniotic membranes in the treatment of non-healing ulcers of different etiologies. Cell Tissue Bank 2004;5(2):129–34.

13. John T. Human amniotic membrane transplantation: past, present and future. Ophthalmol Clin North Am 2003;16:43–65.

14. Niknejad H, Peirovi H, Jorjani M, et al. Properties of the amniotic membrane for potential use in tissue engineering. Eur Cell Mater 2008;15:88–99.

15. Parry S, Strauss JF. Premature rupture of the fetal membrane. N Engl J Med 1998; 338(10):663–70.

16. Adzick NS, Lorenz HP. Cells, matrix, growth factors and the surgeon: the biology of scarless fetal wound repair. Ann Surg 1994;220:10–8.

17. Hao Y, Ma DH, Hwang DG, et al. Identification of antiagiogenic and anti-inflammatory proteins in human amniotic membrane. Cornea 2000;19:348–52.

18. Koob TJ, Rennert R, Zabek N, et al. Biological properties of dehydrated human amnion/chorion composite graft: implications for chronic wound healing. Int Wound J 2013;10:493–500.

19. Schultz GS, Davidson JM, Kirsner RS, et al. Dynamic reciprocity in the wound microenvironment. Wound Repair Regen 2011;19:134–48.

20. Koob TJ, Lim JJ, Zabek N, et al. Cytokines in single layer amnion allografts compared to multi-layered amnion/chorion allografts for wound healing. J Biomed Mater Res B Appl Biomater 2015;103(5):1133–40.

21. Koob TJ, Lim JJ, Massee M, et al. Properties of dehydrated human amnion/chorion composite grafts: implications for wound repair and soft tissue regeneration. J Biomed Mater Res B Appl Biomater 2014;102:1353–62.

22. Koob TJ, Lim JJ, Massee M, et al. Angiogenic properties of dehydrated human amnion/chorion allografts: therapeutic potential for soft tissue repair and regeneration. Vasc Cell 2014;6:10.

23. Chen WY, Abatangelo G. Functions of hyaluronan in wound repair. Wound Repair Regen 1999;7:79–89.

24. Letendre S, LaPorta G, O'Donnell E, et al. Pilot trial of biovance collagen-based wound covering for diabetic ulcers. Adv Skin Wound Care 2009;22:161–6.

25. Zelen CM, Serena TE, Denoziere G, et al. A prospective randomized comparative parallel study of amniotic membrane wound graft in the management of diabetic foot ulcers. Int Wound J 2013;10:502–7.

26. Lavery LA, Fulmer J, Shebetka KA, et al. The efficacy and safety of Grafix for the treatment of chronic diabetic foot ulcers: results of a multi-centre, controlled, randomised, blinded, clinical trial. Int Wound J 2014;11:554–60.

27. DiDomenico LA, Orgill DP, Galiano RD, et al. Aseptically processed placental membrane improves healing of diabetic foot ulcerations: prospective, randomized clinical trial. Plast Reconstr Surg Glob Open 2016;4(10):e1095.

28. Smiell JM, Treadwell T, Hahn HD, et al. Real-world experience with a decellularized dehydrated human amniotic membrane allograft. Wounds 2015;27(6): 158–69.

29. Zelen CM, Serena TE, Gould L, et al. Treatment of chronic diabetic lower extremity ulcers with advanced therapies: a prospective, randomized, controlled, multi-centre comparative study examining clinical efficacy of cost. Int Wound J 2016; 13:272–82.

30. Serena TE, Carter MJ, Le LT, et al. A multicenter, randomized, controlled clinical trial evaluating the use of dehydrated human amnion/chorion membrane allografts and multilayer compression therapy vs. multilayer compression therapy

alone in the treatment of venous leg ulcers. Wound Repair Regen 2014;22: 688–93.
31. Zelen CM. An evaluation of dehydrated human amniotic membrane allografts in patients with DFUs. J Wound Care 2013;10:502–7.
32. Werber B, Martin E. A prospective study of 20 foot and ankle wounds treated with cryopreserved amniotic membrane and fluid allograft. J Foot Ankle Surg 2013;52: 615–21.

The Use of Particulated Juvenile Allograft Cartilage in Foot and Ankle Surgery

Alan Ng, DPM[a,b,]*, Kaitlyn Bernhard, DPM[a]

KEYWORDS

- Particulated juvenile allograft cartilage • Osteochondral lesions of the talus
- Cartilage restoration

KEY POINTS

- Particulated juvenile allograft cartilage (PJAC) has significant promise moving forward and is currently supported by several literature studies.
- Potential benefits of this new technique include single-stage procedure, simplicity in the surgical technique, implantation of juvenile tissue, and a lack of donor site morbidity.
- Since 2012, case series have begun to be published beyond the initial case studies supporting these benefits; however, all but 2 of these focus on chondral lesions of the knee.

INTRODUCTION

Particulated juvenile allograft cartilage (PJAC; DeNovo NT Natural Tissue Graft, Zimmer Inc, Warsaw, Indiana, USA), a regenerative cartilage technology, is intended to treat focal cartilage injuries. Trauma to cartilage of the talus causes osteochondral lesions of the talus (OLT) and can result in pain and loss of function. It is known that adult cartilage has impaired capabilities of intrinsic repair; therefore, symptomatic OLT usually necessitates operative intervention. Other surgical treatments include marrow stimulation, osteochondral autograft or allograft transplantation, micronized allograft cartilage matrix, and autologous chondrocyte implantation; however, that discussion is not in the scope of this article.

Dr Ng is a Consultant in Zimmer/Biomet. Dr Bernhard has nothing to disclose.
[a] PMSR/RRA, Highlands/Presbyterian St. Luke's Podiatric Surgical Residency Program, 1719 East 19th Avenue, Denver, CO 80218, USA; [b] Private Practice, Advanced Orthopedic and Sports Medicine Specialists, 8101 East Lowry Boulevard, #230, Denver, CO 80230, USA
* Corresponding author. PMSR/RRA, Highlands/Presbyterian St. Luke's Podiatric Surgical Residency Program, 1719 East 19th Avenue, Denver, CO 80218.
E-mail address: Ang@advancedortho.org

Clin Podiatr Med Surg 35 (2018) 11–18
http://dx.doi.org/10.1016/j.cpm.2017.08.003
0891-8422/18/© 2017 Elsevier Inc. All rights reserved.

The first reported use of PJAC was in 2007 for the repair of a full-thickness symptomatic patellar chondral defect. Two years after the procedure, the patient demonstrated significant improvement in both pain and function with MRI findings of the defect filled with repair tissue.[1] Application of DeNovo NT to treat isolated cartilage defects has since expanded to the knee, talus, metatarsophalangeal joint, elbow, shoulder, and hip.[2] This article reviews PJAC and its use in foot and ankle surgery.

JUVENILE CARTILAGE BENEFITS

In a controlled laboratory study, it was discovered that human chondrocyte chondrogenic potential declines with age. It was noted that juvenile cells grew significantly faster, they were 100-fold more active in producing cartilaginous tissue than adult counterparts in vitro. In addition, juvenile-derived chondrocytes produced significantly more extracellular matrix compared with chondrocytes from adult donors. The distributions of collagens II and IX were similar in native juvenile cartilage and in neocartilage made by juvenile cells.[3] Although articular cartilage has long been considered immune-privileged, Adkisson and colleagues[4] confirmed that neocartilage derived from juvenile chondrocytes do not stimulate an immunologic response in vivo.

PARTICULATED JUVENILE ALLOGRAFT CARTILAGE

A novel cartilage restoration option, DeNovo NT, has been described using multiple fresh juvenile cartilage allograft tissue pieces, about 1 mm^3 in size, containing scaffold-free living cells within their native extracellular matrix. The allograft is obtained mostly from donors younger than the age of 2 years but can be harvested from neomorts aged younger than 13 years. No stillborn or fetal tissue is used.[5] Each lot consists of multiple packages of PJAC tissue from a single donor and undergoes microorganism testing and standard disease screening in compliance with Good Tissue Practice.[1] An off-the-shelf allograft, it is stored in a sterile medium between 19°C and 26°C. From procurement to expiration date, a package is viable up to 49 days.[6] One package has enough particulated cartilage to fill a 2.5 cm^2 defect.

Imaging Preparation

Although radiographs may appear normal, advanced imaging, such as computed tomography (CT) and MRI are helpful to assess the chondral or osteochondral pathologic condition. MRI has certain advantages compared with CT because it is able to demonstrate bone marrow edema and the stability of the OLT. However, CT is superior in identifying bony structure, especially identifying cystic lesions. Specifically, CT arthrogram is superior to both with its ability to demonstrate very precise analysis of the bone matrix and the cartilaginous cover provided by arthrography.[7]

Indications and Contraindications

An ideal candidate for articular cartilage repair would a focal, unipolar, nondegenerative, full-thickness cartilage defect in younger individuals without uncorrected malalignment. This procedure is recommended in symptomatic articular cartilage, including lesions larger than 15 mm in diameter postdebridement. However, patients with a large lesion, cystic lesion, or previous failed marrow-stimulated procedure are still eligible. Relative indications include shoulder lesions or small

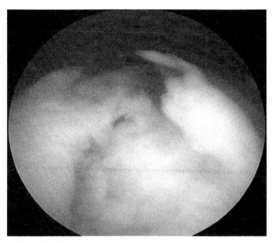

Fig. 1. Large OLT before debridement.

cystic lesions that can be filled and then covered with DeNovo NT. Some contra-indications include large cystic lesions, avascular necrosis, active infections, diffuse arthritis, and osseous malalignment.[8]

Technique

Open versus arthroscopic

Essentially, there are 2 ways to perform a PJAC procedure: open or arthroscopically. Because no literature exists comparing the 2 techniques, the final choice often comes down to location of the injury, size of the lesion, and surgeon preference. No matter the technique, the patient is positioned supine on the operating table. A well-padded thigh tourniquet is applied and inflated to appropriate pressure after exsanguinating the limb. Presented here are the basics of the different procedures.

When performing the procedure arthroscopically, as depicted in **Figs. 1–6**, a standard noninvasive ankle distractor is applied and the anteromedial and anterolateral

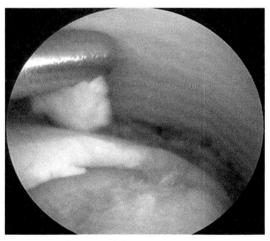

Fig. 2. After arthroscopic debridement of the OLT.

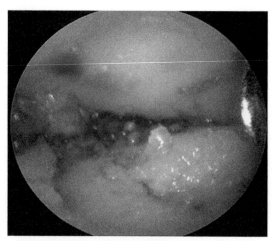

Fig. 3. Drying out of the ankle joint with insufflation.

portals are obtained. The osteochondral lesion is identified and debrided of any overlying fibrocartilage or diseased hyaline cartilage using shavers and curettes. A border of healthy cartilage and intact subchondral bone to provide a lacuna for the PJAC is essential. An abdominal insufflator at 20 mm Hg is used to dry the ankle joint, with suction applied to the second portal, for approximately 5 minutes. Cotton-tip applicators can be used to assist in drying the prepared defect. A layer of fibrin glue is applied. Then the abdominal insufflator is turned off before inserting the PJAC arthroscopically with a 10-g catheter. A small Freer elevator can be used to smooth the PJAC into a single layer covering the cartilaginous defect. A final layer of fibrin glue is applied over the allograft. It is preferred that the subchondral bone is intact, healthy appearing, and dry enough to allow for adhesion of the fibrin glue. If the lesion involves the subchondral plate, as is seen most OLT, it is important to control the bleeding from the osseous bed. Utilization of the fibrin glue can also act as a coagulant to assist in maintaining a blood-free graft bed to prevent any hematoma formation under the

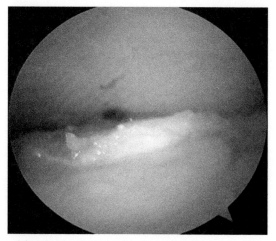

Fig. 4. Application of first layer of fibrin glue to bare OLT.

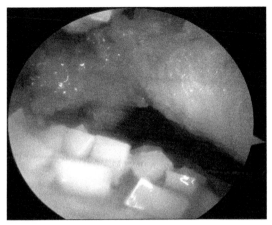

Fig. 5. Application of particulated juvenile allograft to fibrin glue.

anticipated graft site. The PJAC is applied as previously described. The abdominal insufflator is again used to dry the PJAC until the fibrin is firm to the touch. The arthroscopic portals are then closed in standard, layered fashion.[9] An example of the incorporated PJAC at 12 months is shown in **Fig. 7**, which were taken during arthroscopic debridement for a painful ankle impingement.

Alternatively, open procedures have been described for more difficult to reach lesions.[5] Generally, arthroscopy is still performed to remove any synovitis and identify the OLT. Depending on location of the lesion, standard lateral or medial ankle arthrotomies with or without their associated malleolar osteotomies can be performed, as could a plafondplasty for posterior-central lesions. Any of these techniques allows for direct, open visualization of the deficit. Once visualized, there are 2 described ways of applying the PJAC graft. The first method, derived from the technique used in the knee, may not be feasible for still difficult to reach lesions. Taking the sterile,

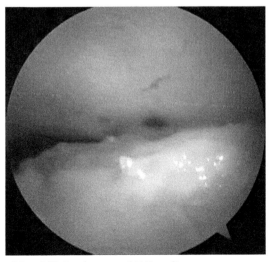

Fig. 6. Final application of fibrin glue over PJAC graft.

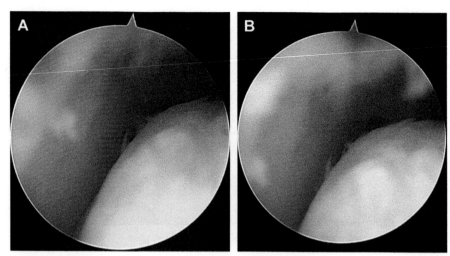

Fig. 7. Twelve-month follow-up of PJAC (*A*). Second look was performed at time of an anterior ankle impingement repair (*B*).

foil lid of the PJAC graft, a 3-dimensional mold is created by press fitting it into the lesion. This mold is then carefully filled with a combination of PJAC and fibrin preparation to create a more structural graft. The graft should not be proud or prominent from the depth of the mold. After 5 to 10 minutes of setting, the graft is transferred to the talus with a base of fibrin glue to the subchondral bone. If the lesion is too difficult to allow creation of an accurate mold, the subchondral bone is covered with a base of fibrin glue, followed by application of the particulated pieces of cartilage graft using a Freer elevator to fill the deficit. Again, the graft should not sit above the adjacent, native cartilage. Fibrin glue is then applied to seal the PJAC graft. Before the graft is completely set, the ankle is dorsiflexed to apply axial force and make the graft more congruous with the remainder of the talar cartilage. The incisions are then closed in standard fashion.

Postoperative Management

To allow for incorporation of the allograft, the patient is kept nonweightbearing for 4 weeks. After 2 weeks, the patient is transitioned into a removable cast boot, remaining nonweightbearing for 2 more weeks but is encouraged to perform range-of-motion activities. At 4 weeks, the patient may progress to full weightbearing in the boot. Starting at week 6, the patients can bear weight in regular shoes and may use a lace-up brace. Physical therapy, strengthening exercises, stationary bicycling, and water activities may be initiated at 6 weeks. The patient should not start impact activities until about 4 to 6 months.[5,9]

SUMMARY

PJAC has significant promise moving forward and is currently supported by several literature studies. Potential benefits of this new technique include single-stage procedure, simplicity in the surgical technique, implantation of juvenile tissue, and a lack of donor site morbidity. Since 2012, case series have begun to be published, beyond the initial case studies supporting these benefits; however, all but 2 of these focus on chondral lesions of the knee.

Bleazey and Brigido[10] collected early results from 7 subjects who underwent repair with a cylindrical sponge allograft, as well as PJAC for cystic OLTs. Using an open procedure, an allograft plug was press fit into the talus and covered with PJAC. Results at 6 months showed no adverse effects to the PJAC or the cylindrical allograft. All subjects reported decreased pain and increased function, despite need for either a tibial or fibular osteotomy in all cases.

Coetzee and colleagues[11] presented data from a case series of 24 ankles treated with PJAC for complicated talar osteochondral lesions. At final follow-up, 78% of subjects had good to excellent results on the American Orthopedic Foot and Ankle Society Score (AOFAS) scale. Of subjects with lesions between 1 and 1.5 cm in maximal dimension, 92% had good to excellent results. Only 1 subject was deemed a failure and suffered from delamination of the graft at 16 months.

One comparative study, published by Lanham and colleagues[12] in 2016, looked at results of PJAC and bone marrow aspirate concentrate (BMAC) with a collagen scaffold for use in OLTs. Six subjects from each treatment were included with similar demographics for each group. At 2 years follow-up, PJAC had a statistically significant improvement compared with BMAC in AOFAS, FAAM (Foot and Ankle Ability Measure) activities of daily living subscale, and FAAM sports subscale scores. The Short Form-12 scores were similar, although when size was accounted for, a trend toward improved outcomes was noted with PJAC in lesions greater than 150 mm^2.

Saltzman and colleagues[13] published a smaller series of 6 ankles treated with PJAC in 2017. Final follow-up was at an average of 13 months and all 6 subjects reported improvements in pain and range of motion. Of note, repeat MRIs were obtained in half of the subjects and all 3 had persistent chondral surface irregularities. These results compared favorably to their systemic review of PJAC, which included only 2 case studies,[9,14] along with the previously mentioned Coetzee and colleagues[11] and Bleazey and Brigido[10] articles.

PJAC is being increasingly studied and has yielded promising results through these few published reports and several isolated case studies. Currently, it has been thoroughly demonstrated that this technique is safe and effective in the short term. Long-term studies are still lacking due to the novelty of the procedure itself. The use of PJAC should increase as an option for cartilage restoration, supported by these early studies and basic science reports.

REFERENCES

1. Bonner K, Daner W, Yao J. 2-year postoperative evaluation of a patient with a symptomatic full-thickness patella cartilage defect repaired with particulated juvenile cartilage tissue. J Knee Surg 2010;23(2):109–14.
2. Cerrato R. Particulated juvenile articular cartilage allograft transplantation for osteochondral lesions of the talus. Foot Ankle Clin N Am 2013;18:79–87.
3. Adkisson H, Martin J, Amendola R, et al. The potential of human allogenic juvenile chondrocytes for restoration of articular cartilage. Am J Sports Med 2010;38(7):1324–33.
4. Adkisson H, Milliman C, Zhang X, et al. Immune evasion by neocartilage-derived chondrocytes: implications for biologic repair of joint articular cartilage. Stem Cell Res 2010;4(1):57–68.
5. Adams S, Easley M, Schon L. Particulated juvenile articular cartilage allograft transplantation for osteochondral lesions of the talus. Oper Tech Orthop 2014;24(3):181–9.

6. Tompkins M, Adkisson D, Bonner K. DeNovo NT. Allograft. Oper Tech Sports Med 2013;21(2):82–9.
7. Laffenetre O. Osteochondral lesions of the talus: current concept. Orthop Traumatol Surg Res 2010;96(5):554–66.
8. Demetracopoulos C, Adams S, Parekh S. Arthroscopic delivery of particulated juvenile cartilage allograft for osteochondral lesions of the talus. Tech Foot Ankle Surg 2014;13(1):39–45.
9. Kruse D, Ng A, Paden M, et al. Arthroscopic De Novo NT juvenile allograft cartilage implantation in the talus: a case presentation. J Foot Ankle Surg 2012;51: 218–21.
10. Bleazey S, Brigido S. Reconstruction of complex osteochondral lesions of the talus with cylindrical sponge allograft and particulate juvenile cartilage graft: provisional results with a short-term follow-up. Foot Ankle Spec 2012;5(5):300–5.
11. Coetzee J, Giza E, Schon L, et al. Treatment of osteochondral lesions of the talus with particulated juvenile cartilage. Foot Ankle Int 2013;34(9):1205–11.
12. Lanham N, Carroll J, Cooper M, et al. A comparison of outcomes of particulated juvenile articular cartilage and bone marrow aspirate concentrate for articular cartilage lesions of the talus. Foot Ankle Spec 2017;10(4):315–21.
13. Saltzman B, Lin J, Lee S. Particulated juvenile articular cartilage allograft transplantation for osteochondral talar lesions. Cartilage 2017;8(1):61–72.
14. Hatic S, Berlet G. Particulated juvenile articular cartilage graft (DeNovo NT Graft) for treatment of osteochondral lesions of the talus. Foot Ankle Spec 2010;3(6): 361–4.

Bone Marrow Aspirate Concentrate and Its Uses in the Foot and Ankle

James M. Cottom, DPM*, Britton S. Plemmons, DPM, AACFAS

KEYWORDS

- BMAC • Regenerative medicine • Bone marrow aspirate • Tendon • Ligament
- Joint • Foot • Ankle

KEY POINTS

- Improving patient outcomes and returning them to their preinjury state is of utmost importance for all foot and ankle surgeons.
- The use of bone marrow aspirate concentrate (BMAC) for augmentation in bone, soft tissue, and chondral repair shows promising results.
- There is a great need for high-level research to further analyze the positive efficacy BMAC on improved outcomes in healing pathologic conditions in the foot and ankle.
- There is little argument that harvesting bone marrow aspirate in the lower extremity is safe and cost-effective with no major complications reported.

INTRODUCTION

Foot and ankle surgeons diagnose and treat a plethora of ailments that can be addressed both conservatively and surgically. Many times, patients wish to avoid the operating room at all costs, whereas others must undergo a surgical procedure to ensure the best prognosis. Because the health care system in the United States continues to evolve and quality measures are driving reimbursement, improving patient outcomes are what every foot and ankle surgeon strives to accomplish. Numerous orthobiologics have been advocated in the orthopedic literature as an adjunct to routine healing to increase the success of a particular treatment regimen. Bone marrow aspirate concentrate (BMAC) has gained popularity, particularly in the foot and ankle subspecialty arena, as an augmentation to healing in and out of the operating room. Unfortunately, patients are often compromised with multiple comorbidities, including diabetes, smoking, compromised immunity, and avascular

The authors have nothing to disclose.
Florida Orthopedic Foot & Ankle Center, 2030 Bee Ridge Road, Suite B, Sarasota, FL 34239, USA
* Corresponding author.
E-mail address: jamescottom300@hotmail.com

necrosis, which may make healing difficult. BMAC use has been widespread and particularly positive results have been seen in bone and soft-tissue healing.[1–5]

BMAC has been used for the adjunctive treatment of numerous pathologic conditions in orthopedics.[6] Viable cells are found in aspiration from many different anatomic regions of the body.[7] Concentration of these cells has been shown to improve healing due to the increased number of certain important cells.[8] There is known benefit from autologous bone marrow concentrate. It has been shown that there is wide variety of live cells, including endothelial progenitor cells, mesenchymal stem cells (MSCs), hematopoietic stem cells (HSCs), and other progenitor cells. There are also many growth factors, including platelet-derived growth factor, bone morphogenic protein, transforming growth factor-B, vascular endothelial growth factor, interleukin (IL)-8, and IL-1 receptor antagonist.[9–14] Bone marrow is the primary site of MSCs, which are multipotent and aid in soft tissue and bone healing.[15–18] MSCs have the innate ability to differentiate into cell types based on the environment. These cellular transitions include fibroblasts, chondrocytes, osteoblasts, and myogenic cells.

The safety of harvesting BMAC has been reported on.[19,20] A complication rate of 0% to 12% has been documented in the harvesting of BMAC in the lower extremity. Bone marrow aspiration from the calcaneus can be performed with ease (**Fig. 1**). Roukis and colleagues[21] performed a multicenter, retrospective, observational cohort study looking at 530 subjects. All subjects underwent harvest of bone marrow aspiration from various sites in the lower extremity. All procedures were determined to be successful with no infection, nerve injury, wound healing, or iatrogenic fractures.

Theoretic evidence of the utility of BMAC to aid in healing has been reported. The authors reviewed the orthopedic and foot and ankle literature to review the uses of BMAC in healing common foot and ankle conditions.

MECHANISM

Recently, there has been a spike in interest in the use of BMAC in the foot and ankle literature. This is because it is a cost-effective way to deliver a conglomerate of stem cells and growth factors to a particular area. Much of the focus on the benefit of BMAC in foot and ankle surgery is on the potential for MSCs to differentiate into different tissue derived from mesenchymal cells. Numerous tissues have been found to contain MSCs, including bone, adipose tissue, synovium, and blood.[22,23] A multitude of

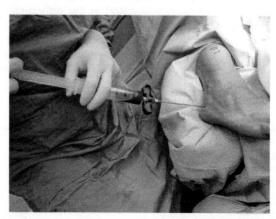

Fig. 1. Intraoperative harvesting of bone marrow aspirate from the calcaneus.

methods have been attempted to harvest, cultivate, and deliver MSCs to an area; many of which accrued a large financial burden. Due to the feasibility of bone marrow aspiration, this method has been researched extensively. BMAC has been proven to yield only 0.001% to 0.01% of the nucleated cells as MSCs. This surprisingly low number has caused researchers to try and enhance the volume of MSCs, most commonly by centrifuge, to reach a concentrate that will yield a higher number of cells. Hegde and colleagues[24] evaluated the efficacy of 3 different BMAC harvesting systems available on the market. Subjects underwent aspiration from bilateral iliac crests using different systems. The aspirate was prepared with the company's proprietary centrifugation system. The Harvest system (Harvest SmartPreP 2, Harvest Terumo BCT, Lakewood, CO, USA) was found to have a significantly greater concentration of progenitor cells compared with the other systems in the study. The method used to harvest the aspiration is also important. The location of the aspiration has been studied and Hernigou and colleagues[25] compared the use of a 10-mL syringe with 50-mL syringe for aspiration of bone marrow. They found a 300% increase in yield of cells in the 10-mL syringe. There was also a higher cell concentration in the in the first mL of the 10-mL syringe compared with the first 5-mL of the 50-mL syringe. This report concluded that a higher cell yield can be gathered with the smaller volume in the smaller syringe. A report by Hyer and colleagues[7] analyzed the concentration of osteogenic progenitor cells from several different anatomic sites. Their report found that the anterior iliac crest had a higher concentration of progenitor cells compared with the distal tibia and calcaneus. They also found that the calcaneus and distal tibial yielded no statistical difference in cells. Interestingly, there was no difference in yield with increased age, smoking, sex, and diabetes. In a recent report on 10 subjects who underwent BMAC from the calcaneus, Li and colleagues[26] found that there were viable MSCs that were able to differentiate into many different cell lineages when the aspirate was analyzed.

BONE HEALING

Certain cells within BMAC (ie, MSCs) have been shown to differentiate into osteoprogenitor cells through induction of local proteins and growth factors wherever they are transplanted. Similar response is created when HSCs are placed in the same environment. Through cell-mediated signaling, other host cells are recruited to the area through cell-to-cell communication. These effects have a positive effect on bone healing. Several animal studies have shown positive results with the use of BMAC in osseous healing. Gianakos and colleagues[27] reviewed the literature regarding long bone healing in animal models and found strong evidence to support the use of BMAC for healing augmentation. The 35 articles reviewed showed a 100% increase in bone formation in BMAC group compared with the control group. In tibia nonunions, Hernigou and colleagues[28] showed that 53 of 60 atrophic nonunions healed with the use of percutaneous transplant of BMAC. Of note, the subjects with the 7 nonunions reported a lower concentration of BMAC than the others, further confirming the theory of better results with higher cell concentration. Several studies using BMAC to aid in healing in the foot and ankle literature have been reported. Adams and colleagues[29] presented a case report of a medial cuneiform stress fracture refractory to conservative treatment that was healed with BMAC placed through the canal of a cannulated screw. With standard postoperative protocol, the fracture healed and was confirmed with postoperative computed tomography scan.

It has been speculated that high-risk patients with multiple comorbidities that have a negative effect on healing rates may benefit from autograft augmentation. In another report, Hernigou and colleagues compared 86 subjects who received iliac crest autograft and 86 subjects who received BMAC augmentation at the site of tibia or fibula nonunion in a diabetic ankle fracture. Thirty-eight percent of diabetics receiving autograft from the iliac crest failed to demonstrate healing; however, 82% of the subjects who received BMAC demonstrated healing at final follow-up. Also noted was the increase in complications at the harvest site in the autograft subject cohort. There was a significant difference in the healing of diabetic ankle fracture nonunions in the BMAC group compared with the iliac crest bone graft group.[30–32] Two studies looked at time to healing in proximal fifth metatarsal fractures fixed with internal fixation and BMAC. One study found healing to be complete at 5 weeks and the other at 7.5 weeks postprocedure. There were a total of 4 refractures in 36 subjects between the 2 reports.

TENDON REPAIR

The mechanisms of tendon injury include mechanical stress, inflammatory process, degenerative changes, and disorganized healing. One theory is to increase the rate of tenocyte proliferation to strengthen the recovery and healing of an injured tendon. One method is to augment tendon healing with BMAC biologic solution. Many mechanisms have been proposed about the actual cellular healing that is provided by BMAC. Cells contained in BMAC can modulate the healing response of pathologic tendon by controlling inflammation, reducing fibrosis, and recruiting other cells, including tenocytes and MSCs. Courneya and colleagues[33] demonstrated that IL-4 and IL-13 were able to stimulate the proliferation of the human tenocyte. The contents of BMAC have been shown to include vascular endothelial growth factor and other cells to aid in healing. It should be considered in augmenting tendon repair because most nontraumatic tendon injuries begin as asymptomatic injuries with a dysvascular component. There is a paucity of information supporting the use of BMAC augmentation in the use of tendon or soft tissue healing in the foot and ankle. Numerous articles looking at animal models support that adding MSCs and other growth factors to a zone of soft tissue injury will aid in the healing and provide superior biomechanical properties of healed tendon.[2,34,35]

Urdzikova and colleagues[35] evaluated rat models that underwent nonoperative treatment of Achilles tendon rupture. Forty subjects underwent nonoperative care without MSC injection and 41 subjects received MSC injection during the postoperative recovery period. An increase in collagen organization, as well as improved vascularization, was found in the group receiving MSC augmentation. Yao and colleagues[34] evaluated the impact of MSC-coated suture to augment Achilles repair in 105 rats. Increased strength was noted compared with standard suture repair at different postoperative follow-up points. Their conclusion was that MSC augmentation may improve early mechanical properties in tendon repair and jumpstart the repair process. Adams and colleagues[2] studied the effects of suture alone, suture plus stem-cell-concentrate injection, or stem cell–loaded suture in the repair of 108 rat Achilles tendon ruptures. At 14-day follow-up, the tendons from the subjects in the suture-alone group had a lower failure load than the other 2 groups. Stein and colleagues[36] reviewed 27 subjects with Achilles rupture who underwent open repair with BMAC augmentation. Mean follow-up was 29.7 plus or minus 6.1 months. Ninety-two percent of subjects returned to their sport at 5.9 plus or minus 1.8 months. There were no reruptures in the cohort.

CHONDRAL HEALING

Evidence suggests that both operative treatment modalities in treating an osteochondral lesion of the talus (OLT), reparative and regenerative techniques, demonstrate good to excellent short-term and midterm clinical outcomes in up to 85% of cases.[37] Nevertheless, the technical difficulty of the operative procedures and the inevitable deterioration of the regenerated or grafted cartilage are of concern.[38–41] Previous studies propose that a combination of mechanical and biological impairments in the injured ankle joint may affect the deterioration, prompting interest in adjuvant modalities that could improve outcomes by addressing some of these deficits. Orthobiologic augmentation with BMAC may increase the longevity of cartilage repair when operatively treating OLT. Its regenerative properties facilitate tissue healing, improving the quality of cartilage by increasing chondroitin sulfate proteoglycan and improving firmness of the repaired cartilage. BMAC also promotes the growth of hyaline cartilage and decreases the amount of fibrocartilage.[4,22,42,43] Although unapproved by the US Food and Drug Administration, BMAC for chondral injury has yielded some promising results. Whether it is used for repair in osteoarthritis, osteochondral lesions, or just chondral lesions, studies that support its use is becoming more widespread. Clinical applications of BMAC for cartilage repair consist of augmentation in microfracture, direct cartilage repair, and injections for osteoarthritis. There is a paucity of long-term studies that solidify the use of BMAC augmentation in the treatment of OLT.[44] Clanton and colleagues[45] reviewed the results of 7 subjects at a mean follow-up of 8.4 months following arthroscopic treatment of OLT with microfracture and a mixture of cartilage extracellular matrix augmented with BMAC. Activities of daily living subscale scores and the Foot and Ankle Disability Index scores both improved significantly at final follow-up. Fortier and colleagues,[4] in an equine knee comparative study of microfracture with or without BMAC augmentation for the treatment of full-thickness cartilage defects, reported improved defect filling, integration of repair tissue, collagen orientation, and increased glycosaminoglycan and type II collagen content in the BMAC group.

SUMMARY

Improving patient outcomes and returning them to their preinjury state is of utmost importance for all foot and ankle surgeons. The use of BMAC for augmentation in bone, soft tissue, and chondral repair shows promising results. There is, however, a great need for high-level research to further analyze the positive efficacy BMAC on improved outcomes in healing pathologic conditions in the foot and ankle. There is little argument that harvesting BMAC in the lower extremity is safe and cost-effective with no major complications reported.

REFERENCES

1. Hartford JS, Dekker TS, Adams SB. Bone marrow aspirate concentration for bone healing in foot and ankle surgery. Foot Ankle Clin N Am 2016;21:839–45.
2. Adams SB Jr, Thorpe MA, Parks BG, et al. Stem cell-bearing suture improves Achilles tendon healing in a rat model. Foot Ankle Int 2014;35(3):293–9.
3. Connolly JF, Guse R, Tiedeman J, et al. Autologous marrow injection as a substitute for operative grafting of tibial nonunions. Clin Orthop Relat Res 1991;266: 259–70.
4. Fortier LA, Potter HG, Rickey EJ, et al. Concentrated bone marrow aspirate improves full-thickness cartilage repair compared with microfracture in the equine model. J Bone Joint Surg Am 2010;92(10):1927–37.
5. Gangji V, De Maertelaer V, Hauzeur JP. Autologous bone marrow cell implantation in the treatment of non-traumatic osteonecrosis of the femoral head: five year follow-up of a prospective controlled study. Bone 2011;49(5):1005–9.

6. Connolly J, Guse R, Lippiello L, et al. Development of an osteogenic bone marrow preparation. J Bone Joint Surg Am 1989;71(5):684–91.

7. Hyer CF, Berlet GC, Bussewitz BW, et al. Quantitative assessment of the yield of osteoblastic connective tissue progenitors in bone marrow aspirate from the iliac crest, tibia, and calcaneus. J Bone Joint Surg Am 2013;95(14):1312–6.

8. Caplan AI. Adult mesenchymal stem cells for tissue engineering versus regenerative medicine. J Cell Physiol 2007;213(2):341–7.

9. DiGiovanni CW, Lin SS, Baumhauer JF, et al. Recombinant human platelet derived growth factor-BB and beta-tricalcium phosphate (rhPDGF-BB/beta-TCP): an alternative to autogenous bone graft. J Bone Joint Surg Am 2013; 95(13):1184–92.

10. Frey C, Halikus NM, Vu-Rose T, et al. A review of ankle arthrodesis: predisposing factors to nonunion. Foot Ankle Int 1994;15(11):581–4.

11. Easley ME, Trnka HJ, Schon LC, et al. Isolated subtalar arthrodesis. J Bone Joint Surg Am 2000;82(5):613–24.

12. O'Connor KM, Johnson JE, McCormick JJ, et al. Clinical and operative factors related to successful revision arthrodesis in the foot and ankle. Foot Ankle Int 2016;37(8):809–15.

13. Jia X, Peters PG, Schon L, et al. The use of platelet-rich plasma in the management of foot and ankle conditions. Oper Tech Sports Med 2011;19:177–84.

14. Schepull T, Kvist J, Norrman H. Autologous platelets have no effect on the healing of human Achilles tendon ruptures: a randomized single-blind study. Am J Sports Med 2011;39:38–47.

15. Yamaguchi Y, Kubo T, Murakami T, et al. Bone marrow cells differentiate into wound myofibroblasts and accelerate the healing of wounds with exposed bones when combined with an occlusive dressing. Br J Dermatol 2005;152(4):616–27.

16. Hernigou PH, Mathieu G, Poignard A, et al. Percutaneous autologous bone-marrow grafting for nonunions: surgical technique. J Bone Joint Surg 2006; 88-A(Suppl 1):322–7.

17. Chong A, Ang A, Goh J, et al. Bone marrow derived mesenchymal stem cells influence early tendon-healing in a rabbit Achilles tendon model. J Bone Joint Surg 2007;89(1):74–81.

18. Muschler G, Boehm C, Easley K. Aspiration to obtain osteoblast progenitor cells from human bone marrow: the influence of aspiration volume. J Bone Joint Surg 1997;79-A(11):1699–709.

19. Schweinberger M, Roukis T. Percutaneous autologous bone-marrow harvest from the calcaneus and proximal tibia: surgical technique. J Foot Ankle Surg 2007; 46(5):411–4.

20. Schade V, Roukis T. Percutaneous bone marrow aspirate and bone graft harvesting techniques in the lower extremity. Clin Podiatr Med Surg 2008;25(4):733–42.

21. Roukis TS, Hyer CF, Philbin TM, et al. Complications associated with autogenous bone marrow aspirate harvest from the lower extremity: an observational cohort study. J Foot Ankle Surg 2009;48(6):668–71.

22. Dominici M, Le Blanc K, Mueller I, et al. Minimal criteria for defining multipotent mesenchymal stromal cells. The International Society for Cellular Therapy position statement. Cytotherapy 2006;8:315–7.

23. Pittenger MF, Mackay AM, Beck SC, et al. Multilineage potential of adult human mesenchymal stem cells. Science 1999;284:143–7.

24. Hegde V, Shonuga O, Ellis S, et al. A prospective comparison of 3 approved systems for autologous bone marrow concentration demonstrated nonequivalency in progenitor cell number and concentration. J Orthop Trauma 2014;28(10):591–8.

25. Hernigou P, Homma Y, Flouzat Lachaniette CH, et al. Benefits of small volume and small syringe for bone marrow aspirations of mesenchymal stem cells. Int Orthop 2013;37(11):2279–87.

26. Li C, Kilpatrick CD, Kenwood SS, et al. Assessment of multipotent mesenchymal stromal cells in bone marrow aspirate from human calcaneus. J Foot Ankle Surg 2017;56(1):42–6.

27. Gianakos A, Ni A, Zambrana L, et al. Bone marrow aspirate concentrate in animal long bone healing: an analysis of basic science evidence. J Orthop Trauma 2016; 30(1):1–9.

28. Hernigou P, Poignard A, Beaujean F. Percutaneous autologous bone-marrow grafting for nonunions. Influence of the number and concentration of progenitor cells. J Bone Joint Surg Am 2005;87(7):1430–7.

29. Adams SB, Lewis JS Jr, Gupta AK, et al. Cannulated screw delivery of bone marrow aspirate concentrate to a stress fracture nonunion: technique tip. Foot Ankle Int 2013;34(5):740–4.

30. Hernigou P, Guissou I, Homma Y, et al. Percutaneous injection of bone marrow mesenchymal stem cells for ankle non-unions decreases complications in patients with diabetes. Int Orthop 2015;39(8):1639–43.

31. Murawski CD, Kennedy JG. Percutaneous internal fixation of proximal fifth metatarsal jones fractures (zones II and III) with Charlotte Carolina screw and bone marrow aspirate concentrate: an outcome study in athletes. Am J Sports Med 2011;39(6):1295–301.

32. O'Malley M, DeSandis B, Allen A, et al. Operative treatment of fifth metatarsal jones fractures (zones II and III) in the NBA. Foot Ankle Int 2016;37(5):488–500.

33. Courneya JP, Luzina IG, Zeller CB, et al. Interleukins 4 and 13 modulate gene expression and promote proliferation of primary human tenocytes. Fibrogenesis Tissue Repair 2010;3:9.

34. Yao J, Woon CY, Behn A, et al. The effect of suture coated with mesenchymal stem cells and bioactive substrate on tendon repair strength in a rat model. J Hand Surg Am 2012;37:1639–45.

35. Urdzikova LM, Sedlacek R, Suchy T, et al. Human multipotent mesenchymal stem cells improve healing after collagenase tendon injury in the rat. Biomed Eng Online 2014;13:42.

36. Stein BE, Stroh DA, Schon LC. Outcomes of acute Ac hilles tendon rupture repair with bone marrow aspirate concentrate augmentation. Int Orthop 2015;39(5): 901–5.

37. Zengerink M, Struijs PA, Tol JL, et al. Treatment of osteochondral lesions of the talus: a systematic review. Knee Surg Sports Traumatol Arthrosc 2010;18(2): 238–46.

38. Robinson DE, Winson IG, Harries WJ, et al. Arthroscopic treatment of osteochondral lesions of the talus. J Bone Joint Surg Br 2003;85(7):989–93.

39. Ferkel RD, Zanotti RM, Komenda GA, et al. Arthroscopic treatment of chronic osteochondral lesions of the talus: long-term results. Am J Sports Med 2008;36(9): 1750–62.

40. Lee KB, Bai LB, Yoon TR, et al. Second-look arthroscopic findings and clinical outcomes after microfracture for osteochondral lesions of the talus. Am J Sports Med 2009;37(1):63S–70S.

41. Becher C, Driessen A, Hess T, et al. Microfracture for chondral defects of the talus: maintenance of early results at midterm follow-up. Knee Surg Sports Traumatol Arthrosc 2010;18(5):656–63.

42. Lanham NS, Carroll JJ, Cooper MT, et al. A comparison of outcomes of particulated juvenile articular cartilage and bone marrow aspirate concentrate for articular cartilage lesions of the talus. Foot Ankle Spec 2016;10(4):315–21.

43. Holton J, Imam M, Ward J, et al. The basic science of bone marrow aspirate concentrate in chondral injuries. Orthop Rev (Padvia) 2016;8(3):6659.

44. Chahla J, Cinque ME, Shon JM, et al. Bone marrow aspirate concentrate for the treatment of osteochondral lesions of the talus: a systematic review of outcomes. J Exp Orthop 2016;3(1):33.

45. Clanton TO, Johnson NS, Matheny LM. Use of cartilage extracellular matrix and bone marrow aspirate concentrate in treatment of osteochondral lesions of the talus. Tech Foot Ankle Surg 2014;13(4):212–20.

Understanding Frontal Plane Correction in Hallux Valgus Repair

W. Bret Smith, DO, MS[a],*, Paul Dayton, DPM, MS[b],
Robert D. Santrock, MD[c], Daniel J. Hatch, DPM[d]

KEYWORDS

- Frontal plane • Hallux valgus • Bunion • Lapiplasty

KEY POINTS

- Understanding the role that frontal/coronal rotation plays in the mechanics of the hallux-abducto-valgus (HAV) deformity and in the radiographic appearance is vital.
- As we begin to understand the more complex 3-dimensional deformity, it will likely push our understanding further.
- Although the initial concepts proposed are a radical challenge to current HAV dogma, classification systems such as this one will ultimately provide an improved understanding of the pathomechanics and pathogenesis of HAV.

INTRODUCTION

The goal of correction of the hallux-abducto-valgus (HAV) deformity should be to position the first metatarsal and metatarsophalangeal (MTP) joint in a position as close to normal anatomy as possible. The current technique that is discussed attempts to correct the deformity at the center of rotational angulation (CORA) in all 3 planes (coronal/frontal, transverse, and sagittal), and is adjustable to the degree of correction in those planes. There are no limitations to this technique based on severity of the hallux valgus angle (HVA) or intermetatarsal angle (IMA). The presence (or absence) of hypermobility, or sagittal plane malalignment, is not a factor in the use of the triplanar correction technique, and it may be used in either condition. This technique is appropriate for all

All authors are paid consultants for Treace Medical Concepts, Inc.
[a] Orthopedics, University of South Carolina, Palmetto Health-USC Orthopedic Center, 104 Saluda Pointe Drive, Lexington, SC 29072, USA; [b] Department of Podiatric Medicine and Surgery, College of Podiatric Medicine and Surgery, Des Moines University, UnityPoint Clinic, Trinity Regional Medical Center, 3200 Grand Avenue, Des Moines, IA 50312, USA; [c] Department of Orthopaedics, West Virginia University, 1 Medical Center Drive, PO Box 9100, Morgantown, WV 26506-9600, USA; [d] Department of Podiatric Medicine and Surgery, North Colorado PMS Residency, 1600 23rd Avenue, Greeley, CO 80634, USA
* Corresponding author.
E-mail address: wbsmithdo@yahoo.com

Clin Podiatr Med Surg 35 (2018) 27–36
http://dx.doi.org/10.1016/j.cpm.2017.08.002
0891-8422/18/© 2017 Elsevier Inc. All rights reserved.

ages as well. Both the adult and adolescent HAV deformities can be corrected via this approach.

The strength of this triplanar technique is the ability to reliably correct all 3 anatomic planes in hallux valgus deformities before committing to a permanent resection of bone. This includes correcting the coronal/frontal plane metatarsal rotation that is present in 87.3% of hallux valgus deformities when examined by weightbearing computed tomography scan.[1] However, the system is adjustable to correct all deformities, from zero rotation to maximum rotation.

This triplanar technique is contraindicated in the case of the unhealthy first MTP joint, or "degenerative bunion." As with other previously described HAV corrective techniques, an arthritic first MTP joint should be addressed by a first MTP joint arthrodesis.

TECHNIQUE

The patient's operative extremity is marked and consent confirmed. For anesthesia, the authors' preference is a regional extremity nerve block performed by the anesthesia team. Once the nerve block has been completed, the patient is taken to the operative suite. The patient is placed on a radiolucent operating room table. A tourniquet is applied to the operative limb, and the limb is prepped and draped in the usual fashion for the operative procedure. The leg is exsanguinated and the tourniquet inflated to the appropriate pressure.

The initial incision is made over the dorsal aspect of the first tarsometatarsal (TMT) joint, just medial to the extensor hallucis longus tendon (**Fig. 1**: initial exposure). It is

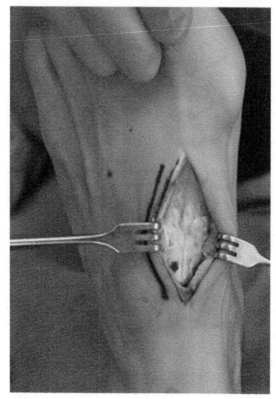

Fig. 1. Dorsal incision.

essential to keep the incision dorsal for this technique to allow the guidance system to work properly. The incision is developed until the dorsal aspect of the first TMT joint is exposed. At this time, the entire dorsal and medial aspects of the joint are subperiosteally dissected.

Next the joint is released to allow for rotation if a frontal plane deformity is noted preoperatively. The joint can be released plantarly using a combination of oscillating saw and osteotome (**Fig. 2**: joint release with osteotome only). A hemostat is then used to open a small space at the proximal aspect of the first and second metatarsal interspace. The fulcrum device (Lapiplasty Fulcrum; Treace Medical Concepts, Ponte Vedra Beach, FL) is then placed into the interspace of the proximal first and second metatarsals (**Fig. 3**: fulcrum placement).

At this time, the mobility of the first MTP joint needs to be evaluated. If it is found to be stiff or ankylosed, then a small webspace incision is made and the tight lateral

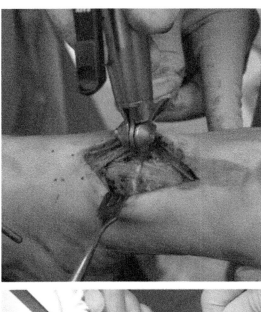

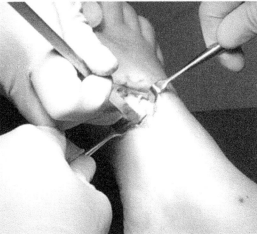

Fig. 2. TMT release (showing both the saw and osteotome options).

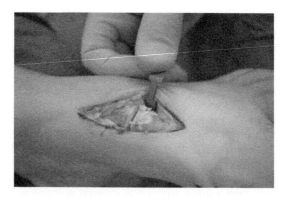

Fig. 3. Fulcrum.

structures are gradually released until the joint is mobilized. It is important to note that you should avoid opening the medial capsule of the first MTP joint at this time because destabilizing the medial structures will not allow the system to correct all 3 planes of the deformity properly.

Once the fulcrum has been placed, a positioner device (Lapiplasty Positioner; Treace Medical Concepts) is ready to be applied. A small stab incision is made over the second metatarsal approximately 1.5 to 2.0 cm distal from the first TMT joint. The positioner is then applied distal to the fulcrum and the joint (**Fig. 4**: positioner placement). The medial aspect of the positioner should be applied to the plantar

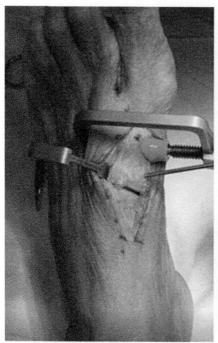
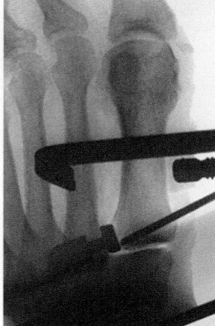

Fig. 4. Positioner (to assist with reduction).

medial ridge on the first metatarsal. The lateral portion of the positioner is placed over the lateral cortex of the second metatarsal.

At this time, the correction of the HAV deformity can be corrected in all 3 planes. Once the correction has been dialed-in to a satisfactory position, it can be confirmed on fluoroscopy. A Kirschner wire can be used to temporarily stabilize the corrected position with a pin placed through a cannulation in the positioner.

A joint seeker (Lapiplasty Joint Seeker; Treace Medical Concepts) is then introduced dorsally in the first TMT joint. This provides a placement guide for the cutting guide (Lapiplasty Cut Guide; Treace Medical Concepts), as well as ensuring that the cuts are made correctly in the sagittal plane to prevent dorsiflexion of the first ray. The cutting guide is then placed and temporarily fixed in place (**Fig. 5**: cutting guide placement). It is recommended at this point to take an image with the c arm to confirm the alignment of the cutting guide. Once the position has been confirmed, a final pin can be introduced to secure the cutting jig in position. The joint seeker is then removed and the cuts on the base of the metatarsal and cuneiform can be completed.

The cut bone is then removed, usually with a combination of osteotome and rongeur. Once all of the cut bone has been removed, the joint is prepared for arthrodesis. A drill bit is used to fenestrate the joint surfaces. At this time, the pin placed through the positioner will need to be removed.

Once the temporary holding pin in the positioner has been removed, the joint is axially compressed and held in the corrected position of choice and precompressed with the terminally threaded olive wire (**Fig. 6**: compression olive wire). A second threaded olive can be placed as well, based on surgeon preference. It is

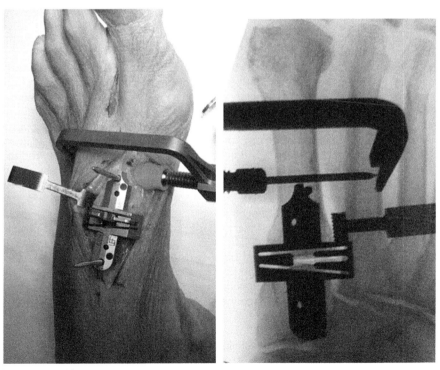

Fig. 5. Cut guide.

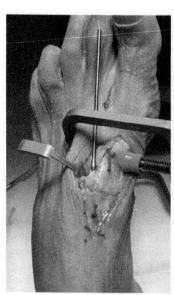
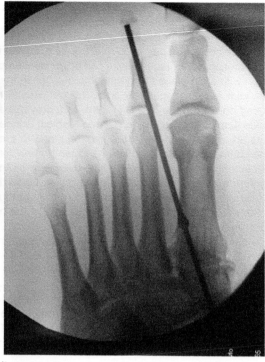

Fig. 6. Olive compression wires holding correction.

recommended at this time to remove or release the positioner and check the correction with fluoroscopy.

If the position is satisfactory, then final fixation can be applied. The current technique uses a biplanar mini-plate construct (Control 360 System; Treace Medical Concepts) that offers stability and allows for physiologic micromotion to promote healing, as described by Perren.[2]

The initial plate is applied straight dorsal across the first TMT joint. Once the plate is positioned, it is temporarily held in position with plate tacks. With the plate held in position, the other open holes are drilled in preparation for screw placement. The drill guides are then removed and the locking screws placed. At this time, the plate tacks can be removed and drill guides and the final 2 locking screws are applied to the plate construct.

At this time, a choice of either a second straight plate can be applied medially across the first TMT joint 90° to the dorsal plate, or a specially designed anatomic plantar-medial–based plate (Plantar Python Plate; Treace Medical Concepts) can be applied. As with the dorsal plate, the second plate is helped with 2 plate tacks and then secured in sequence with the 4 locked screws (**Fig. 7**: plate constructs).

Once the biplanar plate construct has been applied, the surgeon does have the option of adding a screw from the first to the second metatarsal if there is suspicion of intercuneiform instability or if there is a need for additional stabilization of the construct.

Once the first TMT joint has been stabilized, the surgeon can direct his or her attention to the first MTP joint. If needed, a medial-based incision is used to access the joint. Usually, it is noted that there is significant capsular thickening that may require

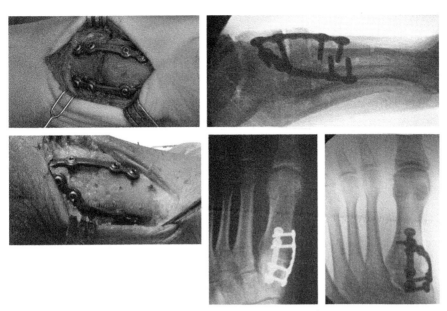

Fig. 7. Plates (demonstrating both biplanar and plantar options).

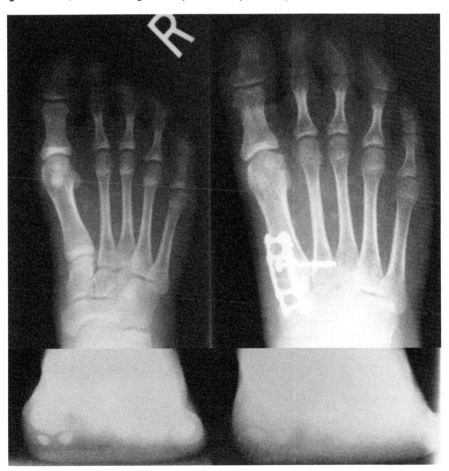

Fig. 8. Note the sesamoid position from rotated to corrected.

thinning. It is also not uncommon to find a dorsal ridge on the first metatarsal head that also may require removal.

Once any additional procedures have been completed, the wounds are copiously irrigated and closed in the standard fashion. The patient is placed into a sterile dressing and either a stiffened postoperative shoe or low walking boot, based on preference.

Several examples are given that represent cases using the triplanar correction technique described in this article (**Figs. 8** and **9**).

DISCUSSION

It is readily evident that the first metatarsal in a bunion is not intrinsically deformed, but it and the hallux are deviated from their normal anatomic alignment.[3,4] When a single osteotomy procedure or, in some cases, more than one osteotomy in the first metatarsal is chosen, new deformities in the metatarsal are created and, at the same time, the original deviation of the metatarsal is not being corrected.[5–7] This practice of creating a surgical deformity of the metatarsal, rather than restoring the normal anatomic alignment, may be one of the reasons for poor outcomes and recurrence.

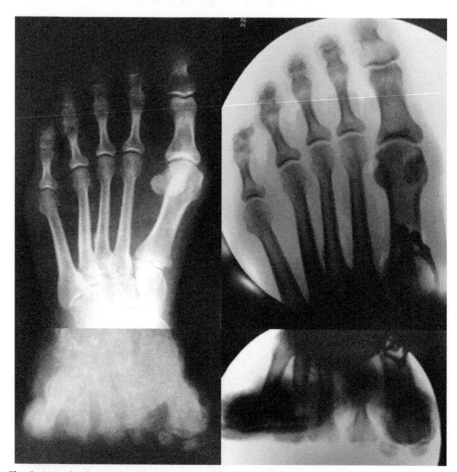

Fig. 9. Note both the derotated metatarsal and realigned sesamoids.

Class	Anatomic Findings	MTP Joint Status	Treatment Recommendation
	Table 1		
	Anatomic triplane HAV classification: new algorithm for approaching treatment of HAV deformity based on 3-dimensional parameters		
1	Increased HVA and IMA *No first metatarsal pronation evident on AP and sesamoid axial radiograph* Sesamoids may be subluxed	No clinical or radiographic evidence of DJD	Transverse plane corrective procedure +/− Distal soft tissue procedures
2A	Increased HVA and IMA *First metatarsal pronation evident on AP and sesamoid axial radiograph* No sesamoid subluxation on axial	No clinical or radiographic evidence of DJD	Triplane correction with first metatarsal supination/ inversion
2B	Increased HVA and IMA *First metatarsal pronation evident on AP and sesamoid axial radiograph* With sesamoid subluxation on axial	No clinical or radiographic evidence of DJD	Triplane correction with first metatarsal supination/ inversion + Distal soft tissue procedures
3	Increased HVA and IMA >15° MTA	No clinical or radiographic evidence of DJD	Metatarsal 2 and 3 transverse plane correction Followed by first metatarsal correction per class 1 and 2 recommendations
4	Increased HVA and IMA +/− First metatarsal pronation	*Clinical and/or radiographic evidence of DJD*	First MTP arthrodesis

Abbreviations: AP, anteroposterior; DJD, degenerative joint disease; HAV, hallux-abducto-valgus; HVA, hallux valgus angle; IMA, intermetatarsal angle; MTA, metatarsus adductus; MTP, metatarsophalangeal.

Recent studies have shown anatomic recurrence rates of up to 78% depending on the procedure studied and, in some cases, the method of measurement used.[8–14] The question at hand is whether these outcomes are due to poor execution of the procedures or to a failure in basic anatomic definition and presurgical classification of the deformities.

For these reasons, it is felt that an improved algorithm should be used when assessing the HAV deformity. This algorithm uses components of all 3 planes of the deformity to drive decision making when approaching bunion correction (**Table 1**).

SUMMARY

We believe that the current paradigm for evaluation of HAV deformity is incomplete. Because it is now understood that recurrence rates with bunion procedures based on traditional algorithms are higher than previously thought and have been linked to uncorrected frontal/coronal plane rotation, it is essential to increase the depth of understanding of this complex 3-dimensional deformity. We propose rethinking the current paradigm for evaluation and management to include all 3 planes of the deformity. Triplane correction of the first metatarsal position ensures the surgeon the flexibility to completely correct the HAV deformity. Understanding the role that frontal/coronal rotation plays in the mechanics of the HAV deformity and in the radiographic appearance is vital. As we begin to understand the more complex 3-dimensional deformity, it will likely push our understanding further. Although the initial concepts proposed are a radical challenge to current HAV dogma, classification systems such as this one will ultimately provide an improved understanding of the pathomechanics and pathogenesis of HAV.

REFERENCES

1. King DM, Toolan BC. Associated deformities and hypermobility in hallux valgus: an investigation with weightbearing radiographs. Foot Ankle Int 2004;25(4): 251–5.
2. Perren SM. Evolution of the internal fixation of long bone fractures. J Bone Joint Surg Br 2002;84:1093–110.
3. Grode SE, McCarthy DJ. The anatomical implications of hallux abducto valgus: a cryomicrotomy study. J Am Podiatry Assoc 1980;70(11):539–51.
4. Thordarson DB, Krewer P. Medial eminence thickness with and without hallux valgus. Foot Ankle Int 2002;23(1):48–50.
5. Tanaka Y, Takakura Y, Kumai T, et al. Radiographic analysis of hallux valgus. J Bone Joint Surg Am 1995;77A(2):205–13.
6. Tanaka Y, Takakura Y, Sugimoto K, et al. Precise anatomic configuration changes in the first ray of the hallux valgus foot. Foot Ankle Int 2000;21(8):651–6.
7. Paley D. Radiographic assessment of lower limb deformities. In: Paley D, editor. Principles of deformity correction. Heidelberg, Germany: Springer; 2002. p. 31–6.
8. Bock P, Kluger R, Kristen K-H, et al. The scarf osteotomy with minimally invasive lateral release for treatment of hallux valgus deformity. J Bone Joint Surg Am 2015;97(15):1238–45.
9. Iyer S, Demetracopoulos CA, Sofka CM, et al. High rate of recurrence following proximal medial opening wedge osteotomy for correction of moderate hallux valgus. Foot Ankle Int 2015;36(7):756–63.
10. Chong A, Nazarian N, Chandrananth J, et al. Surgery for the correction of hallux valgus: minimum five-year results with a validated patient-reported outcome tool and regression analysis. Bone Joint J 2015;97-B(2):208–14.
11. Agrawal Y, Bajaj SK, Flowers MJ. Scarf–Akin osteotomy for hallux valgus in juvenile and adolescent patients. J Pediatr Orthop B 2015;24(6):535–40.
12. Edmonds EW, Ek D, Bomar JD, et al. Preliminary radiographic outcomes of surgical correction in juvenile hallux valgus: single proximal, single distal versus double osteotomies. J Pediatr Orthop 2015;35(3):307–13.
13. Jeuken RM, Schotanus MGM, Kort NP, et al. Long-term follow-up of a randomized controlled trial comparing scarf to chevron osteotomy in hallux valgus correction. Foot Ankle Int 2016;37(7):687–95.
14. Shibuya N, Thorud JC, Martin LR, et al. Evaluation of hallux valgus correction with versus without akin proximal phalanx osteotomy. J Foot Ankle Surg 2016;55(5): 910–4.

Allograft Bone

What Is the Role of Platelet-Derived Growth Factor in Hindfoot and Ankle Fusions

Ryan T. Scott, DPM[a],*, Jeffrey E. McAlister, DPM[a],
Ryan B. Rigby, DPM[b]

KEYWORDS

- Platelet-derived growth factor • PDGF • Ankle • Hindfoot • Fusion • Bone graft
- Allograft

KEY POINTS

- Nonunion is a common complication associated with arthrodesis procedures of the ankle and foot frustrating both patients and surgeons.
- Allograft biologics, such as platelet-derived growth factor (PDGF), are a viable alternative to autogenous bone grafting with reports indicating equivocal outcomes.
- PDGF avoids the obvious morbidity associated with harvesting autogenous bone graft.
- Crushed β-tricalcium phosphate granules are an effective means of delivering PDGF into a fusion site.
- Patients with known risk factors for nonunion should be considered candidates for adjunct biologics such as PDGF.

INTRODUCTION

Biologics have been widely used in ankle and hindfoot arthrodesis for the past several decades. Historically, foot and ankle surgeons have faced significant challenges with regards to achieving a successful arthrodesis. Nonunions also leads to poor patient outcomes, chronic disability, and increased health care expenditure. Literature reports up to a 40% nonunion rate for ankle arthrodesis, 16% for subtalar joint (STJ) arthrodesis, and 17% to 30% for tarsometatarsal joint arthrodesis.[1–4] More recently, a study by Arner and Santrock[5] reports nonunion rates of approximately 10% in ankle and hindfoot fusions. They note a significant increase in nonunion rate associated with smoking, avascular necrosis, and surgical error. Delayed union also remains problematic, especially among patients with known

Disclosure: Dr R.T. Scott is a Consultant for Wright Medical Technologies. Drs J.E. McAlister and R.B. Rigby have nothing to disclose.
[a] The CORE Institute, 18444 North 25th Avenue, Suite 210, Phoenix, AZ 85023, USA; [b] Logan Regional Orthopedics, 1350 North 500 East, Logan, UT 84341, USA
* Corresponding author.
E-mail address: scottryt@gmail.com

Clin Podiatr Med Surg 35 (2018) 37–52
http://dx.doi.org/10.1016/j.cpm.2017.08.008
0891-8422/18/© 2017 Elsevier Inc. All rights reserved.
podiatric.theclinics.com

risk factors. Fortunately, documented rates of tobacco use are declining in the United States; however, diabetes and other clinical risk factors are still prevalent.

Patients with Increased Risk of Nonunion

1. Smokers
2. Diabetics
3. Posttraumatic arthritis
4. Revision surgery
5. Renal impairment

Optimizing arthrodesis rates have brought increased emphasis on mechanical stabilization. Arthroscopic techniques along with new locking plate constructs are attempts to facilitate improved arthrodesis outcomes. However, modern techniques demand biologic augmentation in some patients for increasing surgical success. There are 4 key points in determining the indications for biologics in foot and ankle surgery[6]:

1. What are the specific indications?
2. Where do biologics belong?
3. Which biologics belong?
4. How is this pertinent to my practice?

Once the appropriate patient has been identified for surgery and a biologic is considered, an autograft or allograft is selected. When determining the type of biologic, one should also consider the 3 bone graft properties:

1. Osteoinductive
   a. Direct mesenchymal stem cells (MSCs) to differentiate into osteoblasts
2. Osteoconductive
   a. Provide a scaffold/latticework for new bone formation
3. Osteogenic
   a. Synthesize new bone from within the graft

Although autograft continues to remain the "gold standard," it does carry obvious risks and is not without additional costs. Polly and colleagues[7] demonstrated a significant cost analysis for harvesting iliac crest bone graft (ICBG) during lumbar fusion. The investigators noted the average overall cost of harvesting ICBG to be $2365. Several studies have demonstrated chronic donor site pain and morbidity in harvesting ICBG.[8,9] Schwartz and colleagues[8] noted persistent pain at the donor site to be as high as 25% up to 2 years after surgery. A meta-analysis published by Noshchenko and colleagues[10] found chronic pain of the ICBG site of 49%, nonunion at 24 months at 15%, a 20% rate of major acute complications, and a 7% risk of wound complications. Baumhauer and colleagues[11] in 2013 reviewed 142 patients with bone graft harvest from 5 donor sites: iliac crest, proximal tibia, distal tibia, calcaneus, and other. They concluded that chronic pain was noted in 13% to 20% of bone graft donor sites (proximal tibia < distal tibia < calcaneus).[11,12]

The use of bone marrow aspirate (BMA) added to bone allograft has been an alternative to autologous bone graft harvest.[13] The concept here is to supplement the osteoconductive properties of the demineralized bone matrix with osteoprogenitor cells from the BMA. BMA is typically easy to harvest from multiple sites and carries less morbidity than autologous bone graft harvest. Daigre and colleagues[14] noted there was no significant chronic pain from the BMA harvest in the distal tibia and iliac crest; however, they did find some residual pain from calcaneal BMA. Hyer and colleagues[15] noted the highest concentration of osteoprogenitor cells stemmed from the iliac crest when compared with the tibia and calcaneus. Fitzgibbons and colleagues[16] noted that osteoprogenitor cells in BMAs can be concentrated by use of selective retention systems. These aspirate-matrix composites may be combined with allograft preparations, resulting in a product that promotes osteoconduction, osteoinduction, and osteogenesis with limited morbidity.

The use of rhPDGF-BB may eliminate the need for harvesting BMA in complex hindfoot and ankle surgery.

Platelet-derived growth factor (PDGF) bone graft is indicated for use as an alternative to autograft in arthrodesis of the ankle (tibiotalar joint) or hindfoot (including subtalar, talonavicular, and calcaneocuboid joints, alone or in combination), due to osteoarthritis, posttraumatic arthritis, rheumatoid arthritis, psoriatic arthritis, avascular necrosis, joint instability, joint deformity, congenital defect, or joint arthropathy. PDGF is an option for patients with evidence of a preoperative or intraoperative need for supplemental biologic graft material.[17–21]

Using beta-tricalcium phosphate granules, rhPDGF-BB/β-TCP (Wright Medical Technologies, Memphis, TN) provides an osteoconductive scaffold to deliver the rhPDGF-BB locally. rhPDGF-BB has been demonstrated to carry crucial signaling molecules that stimulate the healing process.[22–29] PDGF-BB plays an important role in stimulating the early phases of bone healing by attracting MSC to the healing environment (chemotaxis), stimulating the rapid division of MSCs (mitogenesis or proliferation).[30,31] PDGF-BB is not a transformation factor, and therefore, does not force MSCs to become a specific type of mature cell. Rather, the large colony of MSCs recruited to the intended fusion site will be stimulated to divide by the locally available differentiation factors. The differentiation is a key detail underlying the overall safety profile of the protein; heterotopic/ectopic bone formation is seen with high-dose exogenous BMPs.

Fiedler and colleagues[32] noted that PDGF has been well documented to recruit cells from surrounding tissue via chemotaxis. PDGF was also noted as a mitogenic agent by recruiting cells to multiply. Bouletreau and colleagues[33] contributed that PDGF upregulates the expression of vascular endothelial growth factor, allowing for angiogenesis. Chemotaxis of MSCs has been noted by rhTGF-B1, rhPDGF, rhBMP-2, rhBMP-4, and rhPDGF-BB.[34] In review of the data from Fiedler and colleagues,[35] it was noted that rhPDGF was 5 times more potent than rhBMP-2.

DiGiovanni and colleagues, in 2013,[36] published a landmark study discussing the utility of rhPDGF-BB in foot and ankle reconstructive surgery. A total of 414 patients treated with hindfoot and ankle arthrodesis were reviewed. Three hundred ninety-seven patients from 37 centers in the United States and Canada were included in the study. The hypothesis of the study was that rhPDGF-BB/β-TCP graft was noninferior to autogenous bone graft. The primary end point was osseous bridging of the arthrodesis site with ≥50% confirmed with computed tomographic (CT) scans. At 24 weeks, those patients who received rhPDGF had comparable healing, CT confirmed, when compared with the autograft group. Clinical healing during this time was noted at 82%. Clinical healing was once again reviewed at 52 weeks. There was no clinical significance in the P value for the rhPDGF group when compared with the autograft group. Clinical healing was 86%. The only clinical significance noted during the study at 52 weeks was chronic graft site pain. The investigators established that rhPDGF-BB/β-TCP was equivalent in clinical outcome and performance when compared with autologous bone graft. They concluded that rhPDGF-BB/β-TCP is a safe and effective alternative to autologous bone graft in hindfoot and ankle arthrodesis.[36–41]

SURGICAL TECHNIQUE

The β-TCP granules may be crushed with a bone tamp to help absorb the rhPDGF. The mixture of rhPDGF included contains 0.3 mg/mL. The PDGF is then added to the β-TCP and allowed to absorb for roughly 10 minutes before implantation. It is recommended that the graft be inserted within 1 hour to ensure maximal benefit. Standard arthrodesis preparation of the joint is performed by removing the cartilaginous surface. The subchondral bone is then fenestrated and fish scaled to allow portals through the subchondral bone. The soaked granules are then packed in the perforations and under any feathering of the cortical bone. Any remaining liquid may be drawn into a syringe and placed into the anticipated arthrodesis site. Remaining deficits are then packed with bone graft. Final irrigation should be performed before rhPDGF implantation.

Over time, the β-TCP is intended to be resorbed at the fusion site and replaced by new bone. Under such circumstances, it would typically be indistinguishable from surrounding bone. The β-TCP component is radiopaque, which must be considered when evaluating radiographs for the assessment of bridging bone, and for this reason, the authors advocate follow-up CT scans at regular intervals.

INDICATIONS

1. Ankle arthrodesis
2. STJ arthrodesis
3. Talonavicular joint arthrodesis
4. Calcaneocuboid joint arthrodesis

CONTRAINDICATIONS

1. Patients who have a known hypersensitivity to any of the components of the product or are allergic to yeast-derived products
2. Patients with active cancer
3. Patients who are skeletally immature (<18 years of age or no radiographic evidence of closure of epiphyses)
4. Pregnant women
5. Patients with an active infection at the operative site
6. Patients with inadequate soft tissue coverage
7. Patients with metabolic disorders known to adversely affect the skeleton (eg, renal osteodystrophy or hypercalcemia), other than primary osteoporosis or diabetes
8. Patients with a substitute for structural graft

As with all therapeutic recombinant proteins, there is a potential for immune responses to be generated to the rhPDGF-BB component. The detection of antibody formation is highly dependent on the sensitivity and specificity of the assay. In addition, the observed incidence of antibody (including neutralizing antibody) positivity in an assay may be influenced by several factors, including assay methodology, sample handling, timing of sample collection, concomitant medications, and underlying disease.

CLINICAL EVALUATION
Case 1

Case 1 was a 44-year-old woman with painful posttraumatic severe ankle arthrosis (**Figs. 1** and **2**). The patient had failed years of conservative treatment. No significant frontal plane malalignment was apparent; however, on the lateral radiograph, the talus was found to have posterior translation. The patient was too young for a total ankle

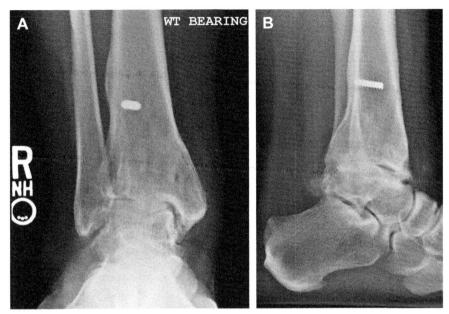

Fig. 1. (*A, B*) Anteroposterior (AP) and lateral radiograph of a 44-year-old with severe post-traumatic arthritis.

replacement and elected for ankle arthrodesis. After obtaining both MRI and CT scans, the patient was deemed a good candidate for arthroscopic ankle fusion. The joint was prepared for fusion arthroscopically, and before placement of the final hardware, PDGF was injected into the fusion site. Initial and final radiographs demonstrate excellent

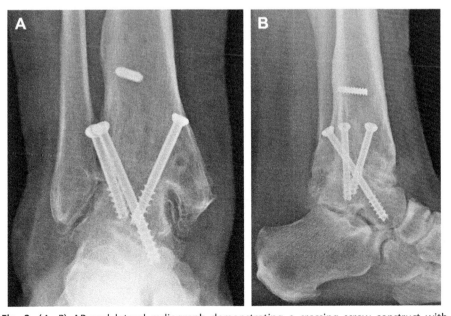

Fig. 2. (*A, B*) AP and lateral radiograph demonstrating a crossing screw construct with osseous union of the tibiotalar joint with augmentation using rh-PDGF.

consolidation of the ankle fusion. The patient was allowed protected weight-bearing beginning at 9 weeks postoperatively and later advanced into regular shoe gear.

Case 2

Case 2 was a 67-year-old man who presented with severe ankle degeneration and longstanding ankle pain and deformity (**Figs. 3–5**). The patient's comorbidities included type 2 diabetes and hypertension. No significant sensory neuropathy was identified. The patient did have valgus malalignment in the frontal plane, however no sagittal plane deformity. No history of ulcerations or infection was reported. The patient failed multiple attempts at conservative treatments and elected for ankle fusion. An anterior incisional approach was performed, and the valgus deformity was reduced. After adequate joint preparation was performed, an anterior locking plate was used. However, before hardware placement, rhPDGF/β-TCP was introduced into the fusion site. Initial and final postoperative radiographs show a well-consolidated, well-aligned arthrodesis. Weight-bearing was allowed at 9 weeks postoperatively.

Case 3

Case 3 was a 66-year-old man who presented complaining of long-term ankle pain (**Figs. 6–9**). The patient reported having a fusion surgery 4 years previously. Radiographs of the ankle demonstrated hardware present across the STJ, and both lateral and calcaneal axial views were suspicious for nonunion. Laboratory markers were negative, and diagnostic block into the STJ region provided significant but only temporary relief. A CT scan was obtained confirming complete nonunion of the STJ. The patient elected for a revision-type procedure. The hardware was removed, and the nonunion was resected with subsequent joint preparation. Before hardware placement, bone graft was performed and rhPDGF/β-TCP was inserted. Final radiographic

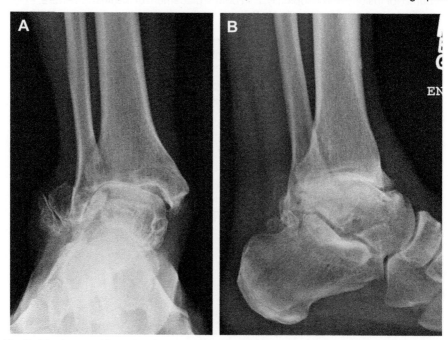

Fig. 3. (*A, B*) AP and lateral radiograph of a 67-year-old with severe posttraumatic arthritis and incongruent ankle valgus.

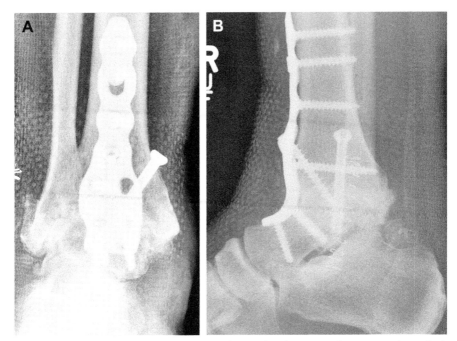

Fig. 4. (*A*, *B*) Immediate postoperative radiographs demonstrating restoration of the anatomic ankle joint with plate fixation for tibiotalar arthrodesis.

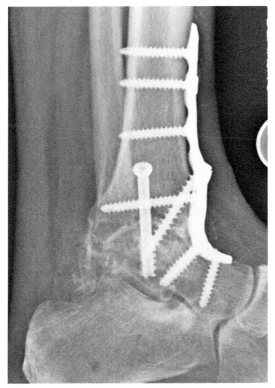

Fig. 5. Osseous union of the tibiotalar joint with plate construct and rh-PDGF at 12 weeks postoperatively.

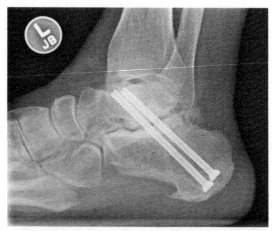

Fig. 6. Lateral radiograph shows nonunion of the posterior facet of the STJ with 2 cannulated compression screws.

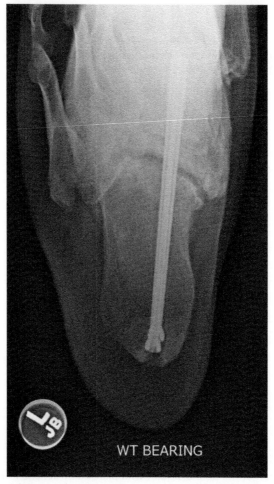

WT BEARING

Fig. 7. Calcaneal axial view redemonstrating nonunion of the posterior facet of the STJ.

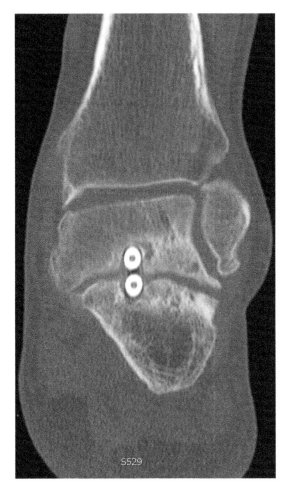

Fig. 8. CT scan shows no osseous bridging of the posterior STJ.

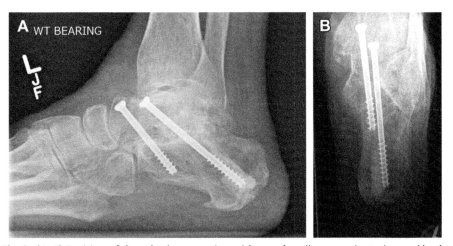

Fig. 9. (*A, B*) Revision of the subtalar nonunion with a push pull screw orientation and back-fill of the previous cannulated screw tracts. Revision was augmented with rh-PDGF.

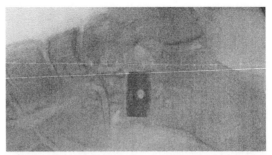

Fig. 10. Patient with previously failed Evans calcaneal osteotomy with trabecular metal construct. (*Courtesy of* Carroll Jones, MD, OrthoCarolina, Charlotte, NC.)

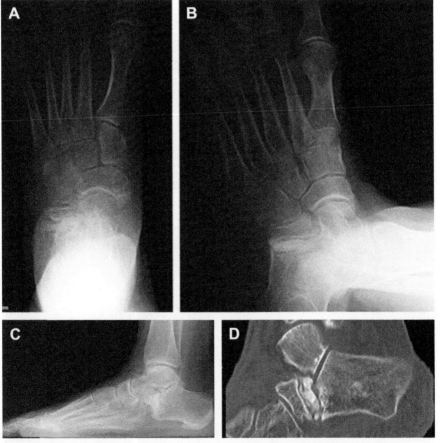

Fig. 11. (*A–D*) Continued nonunion of Evans calcaneal osteotomy following removal of the trabecular metal and conversion to bulk allograft. (*Courtesy of* Carroll Jones, MD, OrthoCarolina, Charlotte, NC.)

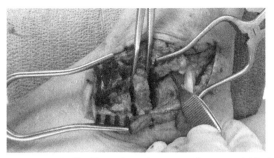

Fig. 12. Resection of retained bulk allograft and surrounding nonviable bone. (*Courtesy of* Carroll Jones, MD, OrthoCarolina, Charlotte, NC.)

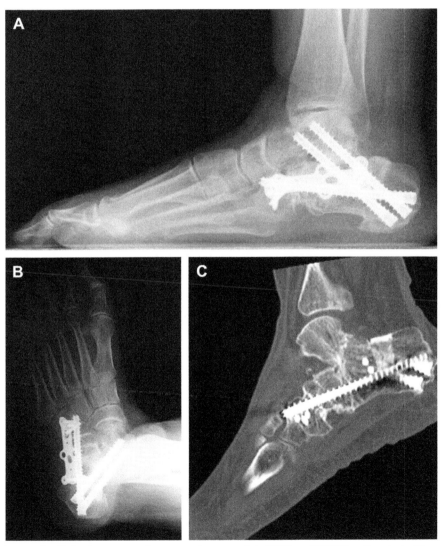

Fig. 13. (*A–C*) Final construct demonstrating use of rh-PDGF and STJ/CCJ arthrodesis. (*Courtesy of* Carroll Jones, MD, OrthoCarolina, Charlotte, NC.)

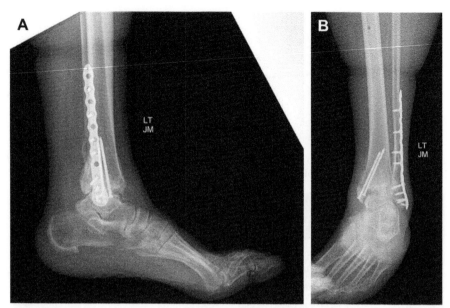

Fig. 14. (*A*, *B*) A 51-year-old with chronic posttraumatic arthritis and nonunion of the medial malleolus.

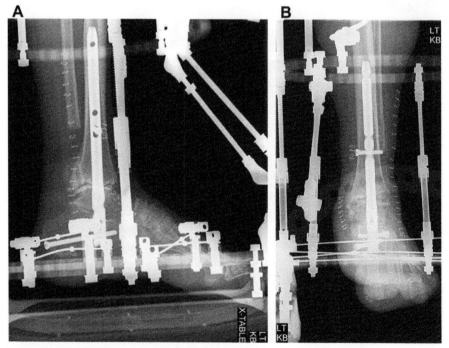

Fig. 15. (*A*, *B*) Immediate postoperative films of hardware removal with fibular osteotomy and a TTC arthrodesis with intramedullary nail, external fixator, and rh-PDGF.

examination demonstrates a well-consolidated STJ. Weight-bearing was allowed at 10 weeks postoperatively.

Case 4

Case 4 was a 50-year-old man with lateral column pain who presented for a third opinion. The patient smokes 1 pack of cigarettes per day (**Figs. 10–13**). The patient has had a previous lateral column-lengthening calcaneal osteotomy with allograft in 2012, revised to trabecular metal in 2014, revised again to allograft and plate fixation. The plate was subsequently removed in 2015 secondary to osteoarthritis. Based on the deficit, a structural autograft was harvested from the posterior superior calcaneus. The Evans calcaneal osteotomy was revised with rhPDGF/β-TCP, calcaneal autograft, as well as a calcanealcuboid (CCJ) and STJ arthrodesis for further stabilization. Final radiographs and CT confirm osseous union of the STJ and CCJ arthrodesis, and the Evans calcaneal osteotomy.

Case 5

Case 5 was a 51-year-old woman with a history of bilateral ankle open reduction, and internal fixation 3 years before, who complained of ongoing left ankle pain (**Figs. 14–16**). Her past medical history included morbid obesity, uncontrolled diabetes

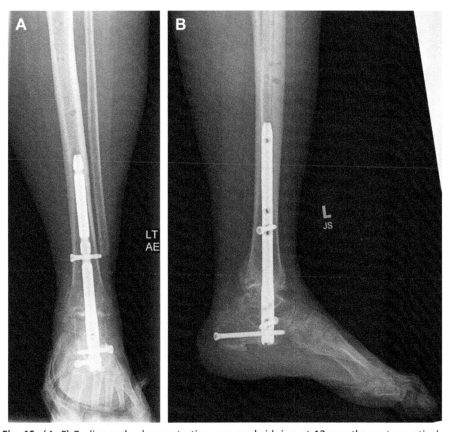

Fig. 16. (A, B) Radiographs demonstrating osseous bridging at 12 months postoperatively.

mellitus, tobacco use, impaired renal function, as well as peripheral neuropathy. Bracing options failed, and tibiotalar joint injections provided short-term relief. Surgical interventions were offered, and because of her high risk of an amputation, a load-sharing device and bone grafting option were consented for tibiotalocalcaneal (TTC) joint fusion with intramedullary fixation. The intraoperative plan was executed without complication, and a TTC was performed with rhPDGF-BB because of her high risk of nonunion. Postoperative radiographs reveal an intramedullary nail with the use of a static external fixator. Postoperative protocol was followed accordingly, and the patient was non-weight-bearing for 2 months. Serial radiographs were taken for osseous healing. At her 1 year follow-up, the patient had clinical and radiographic evidence of a healed TTC fusion. She was weight-bearing without pain in a diabetic shoe.

SUMMARY

As the incidence of foot and ankle nonunion rates increase, the use of biologics in foot and ankle arthrodesis has followed. Historically, ICBG was harvested for use in more complex cases. The literature supports improved union rates with ICBG; however, it also raises cost and pain ramifications. With this being noted, alternative biologics may be considered. PDGF-BB has been shown to provide a safe and successful alternative to harvesting autograft.

ACKNOWLEDGMENTS

Thank you to Dr Carroll Jones (OrthoCarolina, Charlotte, NC) for permission to publish his experience on the use of rhPDGF/β-TCP in hindfoot and ankle arthrodesis.

REFERENCES

1. Frey C, Halikus NM, Vu-Rose T, et al. A review of ankle arthrodesis: predisposing factors to nonunion. Foot Ankle Int 1994;15:581–4.
2. Scranton PE. Use of internal compression in arthrodesis of the ankle. J Bone Joint Surg Am 1985;67(4):550–5.
3. Easley ME, Trnka HJ, Schon LC, et al. Isolated subtalar arthrodesis. J Bone Joint Surg Am 2000;82(5):613–24.
4. Glazebrook M, Beasley W, Daniels T, et al. Establishing the relationship between clinical outcome and extent of osseous bridging between computed tomography assessment in isolated hindfoot and ankle fusions. Foot Ankle Int 2013;34(12): 1612–8.
5. Arner JW, Santrock RD. A historical review of common bone graft materials in foot and ankle surgery. Foot Ankle Spec 2014;7(2):143–51.
6. Lin SS, Montemurro NJ, Krell ES. Orthobiologics in foot and ankle surgery. J Am Acad Orthop Surg 2016;24:113–22.
7. Polly DW Jr, Ackerman SJ, Shaffrey CI, et al. A cost analysis of bone morphogenetic protein versus autogenous iliac crest bone graft in single-level anterior lumbar fusion. Orthopedics 2003;26(10):1027–37.
8. Schwartz CE, Martha JF, Kowalski P, et al. Prospective evaluation of chronic pain associated with posterior autologous iliac crest bone graft harvest and its effect on postoperative outcome. Health Qual Life Outcomes 2009;7:49.
9. Chen YC, Chen CH, Chen PL, et al. Donor site morbidity after harvesting of proximal tibial bone. Head Neck 2006;28(6):496–500.

10. Noshchenko A, Hoffecker L, Lindley EM, et al. Long-term treatment effects of lumbar arthrodesis in degenerative disease: a systematic review with meta-analysis. J Spinal Disord Tech 2015;28(9):E493–521.

11. Baumhauer JF, Pinzur MS, Daniels TR, et al. Survey on the need for bone graft in foot and ankle fusion surgery. Foot Ankle Int 2013;34(12):1629–33.

12. Baumhauer J, Pinzur MS, Donahue R, et al. Site selection and pain outcome after autologous bone graft harvest. Foot Ankle Int 2013;35(2):104–7.

13. Ozaki Y, Nishimura M, Sekiya K, et al. Comprehensive analysis of chemotactic factors for bone marrow mesenchymal stem cells. Stem Cells Dev 2007;16(1):119–29.

14. Dalgro JL, DeMill SI, Hyer CF. Assessment of bone marrow aspiration site pain in foot and ankle surgery. Foot Ankle Spec 2016;9(3):215–7.

15. Hyer CF, Berlet GC, Bussewitz BW, et al. Quantitative assessment of the yield of osteoblastic connective progenitors in bone marrow aspirate from the iliac crest, tibia, calcaneus. J Bone Joint Surg Am 2013;95(14):1312–6.

16. Fitzgibbons TC, Hawkins MA, McMullen ST, et al. Bone grafting in surgery about the foot and ankle: indications and techniques. J Am Aca Orthop Surg 2011;19(2):112–20.

17. Solchaga LA, Daniels T, Roach S, et al. Effect of implantation of Augment(®) bone graft on serum concentrations of platelet-derived growth factors: a pharmacokinetic study. Clin Drug Investig 2013;33(2):143–9.

18. Glazebrook M, Daniels TR, Abidi NA, et al. Role of platelet-derived growth factor in hindfoot fusion. Tech Foot Ankle Surg 2012;11(1):34–8.

19. Solchaga LA, Hee CK, Roach S, et al. Safety of recombinant human platelet-derived growth factor-BB in AUGMENT® Bone Graft. J Tissue Eng 2012;3(1). 2041731412442668.

20. Friedlaender GE, Lin S, Solchaga LA, et al. The role of recombinant human platelet-derived growth factor-BB (rhPDGF-BB) in orthopaedic bone repair and regeneration. Curr Pharm Des 2013;19(19):3384–90.

21. Nevins M, Giannobile WV, McGuire MK, et al. Platelet-derived growth factor stimulates bone ll and rate of attachment level gain: results of a large multicenter randomized controlled trial. J Periodontal 2005;76(12):2205–15.

22. Pountos I, Georgouli T, Henshaw K, et al. The effect of bone morphogenetic protein-2, bone morphogenetic protein-7, parathyroid hormone, and platelet-derived growth factor on the proliferation and osteogenic differentiation of mesenchymal stem cells derived from osteoporotic bone. J Orthop Trauma 2010;24(9):552–6.

23. Moore DC, Ehrlich MG, McAllister SC, et al. Recombinant human platelet-derived growth factor-BB augmentation of new-bone formation in a rat model of distraction osteogenesis. J Bone Joint Surg Am 2009;91(8):1973–84.

24. Al-Zube L, Breitbart EA, O'Connor JP, et al. Recombinant human platelet-derived growth factor BB (rhPDGF-BB) and beta-tricalcium phosphate/collagen matrix enhance fracture healing in a diabetic rat model. J Orthop Res 2009;27(8):1074–81.

25. McCarthy HS, Williams JH, Davie MW, et al. Platelet-derived growth factor stimulates osteoprotegerin production in osteoblastic cells. J Cell Physiol 2009;218(2):350–4.

26. Tokunaga A, Oya T, Ishii Y, et al. PDGF receptor beta is a potent regulator of mesenchymal stromal cell function. J Bone Miner Res 2008;23(9):1519–28.

27. Mehrotra M, Krane SM, Walters K, et al. Differential regulation of platelet-derived growth factor stimulated migration and proliferation in osteoblastic cells. J Cell Biochem 2004;93(4):741–52.
28. Kilian O, Flesch I, Wenisch S, et al. Effects of platelet growth factors on human mesenchymal stem cells and human endothelial cells in vitro. Eur J Med Res 2004;9(7):337–44.
29. Zhang Z, Chen J, Jin D. Platelet-derived growth factor (PDGF)-BB stimulates osteoclastic bone resorption directly: the role of receptor beta. Biochem Biophys Res Commun 1998;251(1):190–4.
30. Hollinger JO, Hart CE, Hirsch SN, et al. Recombinant human platelet-derived growth factor: biology and clinical applications. J Bone Joint Surg Am 2008; 90(Suppl 1):48–54.
31. Hollinger JO, Onikepe AO, MacKrell J, et al. Accelerated fracture healing in the geriatric, osteoporotic rat with recombinant human platelet-derived growth factor-BB and an injectable beta-tricalcium phosphate/collagen matrix. J Orthop Res 2008;26(1):83–90.
32. Fiedler J, Röderer G, Günther KP, et al. BMP-2, BMP-4, and PDGF-bb stimulate chemotactic migration of primary human mesenchymal progenitor cells. J Cell Biochem 2002;87(3):305–12.
33. Bouletreau PJ, Warren SM, Spector JA, et al. Factors in the fracture microenvironment induce primary osteoblast angiogenic cytokine production. Plast Reconstr Surg 2002;110(1):139–48.
34. Kilian O, Alt V, Heiss C, et al. New blood vessel formation and expression of VEGF receptors after implantation of platelet growth factor-enriched biodegradable nanocrystalline hydroxyapatite. Growth Factors 2005;23(2):125–33.
35. Fiedler J, Etzel N, Brenner RE. To go or not to go: migration of human mesenchymal progenitor cells stimulated by isoforms of PDGF. J Cell Biochem 2004; 93(5):990–8.
36. DiGiovanni CW, Lin S, Baumhauer JF, et al. Recombinant human platelet-derived growth factor-BB and beta-tricalcium phosphate (rhPDGF-BB/β-TCP): an alternative to autogenous bone graft. J Bone Joint Surg Am 2013;95(13):1184–92.
37. DiGiovanni CW, Lin SS, Daniels TR, et al. The importance of sufficient graft material in achieving foot or ankle fusion. J Bone Joint Surg Am 2016;98(15):1260–7.
38. DiGiovanni CW, Lin S, Pinzur M. Recombinant human PDGF-BB in foot and ankle fusion. Expert Rev Med Devices 2012;9(2):111–22.
39. DiGiovanni CW, Baumhauer J, Lin SS, et al. Prospective, randomized, multi-center feasibility trial of rhPDGF-BB versus autologous bone graft in a foot and ankle fusion model. Foot Ankle Int 2011;32(4):344–54.
40. DiGiovanni CW, Petricek JM. The evolution of rhPDGF-BB in musculoskeletal repair and its role in foot and ankle fusion surgery. Foot Ankle Clin 2010;15(4): 621–40.
41. Daniels T, DiGiovanni C, Lau JT, et al. Prospective clinical pilot trial in a single cohort group of rhPDGF in foot arthrodesis. Foot Ankle Int 2010;31(6):473–9.

Advancements in Bone Fixation Utilizing Novel Biointegrative Fixation Technology

Bob Baravarian, DPM[a],*, Tal Pnina Lindner, PhD[b],
Ronit Merchav-Feuermann, DVM[c]

KEYWORDS

- Bone • Fixation • Orthopedics • Absorbable • Biocomposite • Biointegrative
- Reinforced • Polymer

KEY POINTS

- Advancement in orthopedics has been increasing rapidly.
- With time, metallic hardware will begin to be replaced by novel materials that become one with the body.
- This progress will not only aid in the repair process it will allow permanent and improved reinforcement of the fixated region.
- Biointegrative technology is a promising new generation of materials capable of achieving this goal.
- It is expected that plates, screws, pins, interference screws, and even possibly joint replacements will incorporate into the patients' bodies, negating the need for hardware removal and adding structure and stability to an iatrogenically weakened area.

INTRODUCTION

Fixation of fractures and osteotomies has progressed dramatically with the advent of internal fixation. Before internal fixation, most fractures were placed in casts and anatomic fixation was difficult to achieve. In the mid-1950s, screw fixation was introduced by the AO Foundation with carpentry techniques used to fixate bone. Over the course of 60 years, fixation has been advanced to include cannulated systems, headless systems, different plate/screw combinations, and some absorbable or allograft

Disclosure: Dr B. Baravarian is an investor in Ossio, head of the foot and ankle advisory board, and a consultant to the company.
[a] UCLA School of Medicine, University Foot and Ankle Institute, Los Angeles, CA 90095, USA;
[b] Scientific and Regulatory Affairs, Ossio Ltd, 58 Hatachana Street, Tel Aviv 3052643, Israel;
[c] Ossio Ltd, 58 Hatachana Street, Tel Aviv 3052643, Israel
* Corresponding author.
E-mail address: BBaravarian@mednet.ucla.edu

bone fixation options. However, there has been little advancement that has dramatically and significantly changed fixation techniques from a biomaterial standpoint, with the main material used still being nonabsorbable steel or titanium.

Metal, in any form, is an excellent fixation material. However, metal has downsides. On a positive note, metal is inert and does not cause much reaction as long as the patient does not have a metal allergy. Second, it offers a solid fixation that is stronger than bone and adds significant strength to a fracture or osteotomy fixation.

On the negative side, metal screws may need to be removed and the AO Foundation recommends removal of hardware, which requires a second surgery. Metal also is not good for imaging and often gives off significant signal with both MRI and computed tomography imaging. In addition, hardware removal may be difficult, with screw stripping and breakage, and can leave the bone hollow in the region of hardware removal, resulting in bone weakness.

Absorbable hardware has been attempted several times in orthopedic fixation. Most of the material previously used was made out of suture material stranded together. The problem with absorbable material has been that the absorption usually occurs all at once with what is called a burst effect, which means that the material degrades significantly and all at once through an acidic process causing cystic changes and leaving the bone exposed to weakness in the region of absorption. Furthermore, the region of absorption has, at times, formed cystic changes that can be painful and grow with time within the bone. In addition, there has been no absorbable material, other than bone, that has offered support and adjustable strength. Such a material would be ideal because it would allow the transfer of strength to the bone slowly while the material is replaced by new bone formation for added strength and stability.

Bone allograft has become popular in foot and ankle fixation. The bone is milled into the shape of pins and plugs that are press fitted into the bone. This technique offers superior benefits to previous absorbable materials because bone can grow into the allograft and allow additional stability; bone allograft rarely needs to be removed; can be cut through, which allows ease of secondary surgery options; and is fairly inert. However, bone allografts have sterility and infection risks. The bone materials also differ in strength depending on the quality of the allograft material, which may differ from person to person. Bone pins or screws also cannot be modified for surgical location–specific strength and absorption options. In addition, the bone material can be brittle during insertion, resulting in fracture or stripping of the hardware during insertion. This risk means that the bone is mainly used as a plug or pin and cannot offer rigid fixation or compression.

THE IDEAL BONE FIXATION MATERIAL

In an ideal situation, fixation of bone should offer multiple benefits and reduce multiple current negative factors. The benefits include:

1. Strength comparable with or greater than the bone that is being fixated, with slow decrease in strength to allow the bone to increase its strength.
2. Absorption of the material in a timely and quiescent manner without burst effect.
3. Replacement of the fixation material with bone to allow for strength, and negate the risk of cysts or hollow bone regions in a slow and sustained manner.
4. Ability to achieve rigid fixation and compression from the material, with multiple forms of fixation being possible in the form of screws, plates, pins, and rods.
5. No need for removal of the material.

If all of these qualities were to be met, absorbable fixation would be superior to nonabsorbable fixation because there would be all the benefits of metal fixation with additional benefits of an ideal absorbable material. If the ideal material could then be further advanced, there would be the added benefits of a material that degrades adequately, allowing the surrounding bone to acquire more strength in a timely manner that could be adjusted for time based on how long each bone and region needs to be protected, and that could also encourage new bone growth in the region of fixation, which would strengthen the bone that is being fixated. Essentially, what is needed is a material that stabilizes the bone with rigid fixation, absorbs gradually, allows the body grow bone in its place, and acts like a bone graft strut in the region of fixation. Ambrose and Clanton[1] noted that, in addition to the information discussed earlier, the degradation of absorbable implants can allow a gradual transference of load from the implant to the bone, thus stimulating robust bone healing.

PREVIOUS MATERIALS AND WHY THEY FAILED

Polylactic acid (PLA) and polyglycolic acid (PGA) and their copolymers have historically been among the most commonly used bioabsorbable polymers in orthopedic implants. Additional polymers, including poly[ortho esters], poly[glycolide-co-trimethylene carbonate], poly[dioxanone], poly[e-caprolactone], and poly[b-hydroxybutyrate] implants are also available. However, most of the commercially available implants are still made of PGA and PLA or their copolymers. These bioabsorbable polymer devices are manufactured in the form of pins, screws, plates, rods, tacks, and suture anchors.

PGA is hydrophilic and highly crystalline. Degradation and strength loss occur early and lead to postoperative complications. PLA is more hydrophobic. Two isomers of PLA, the L-isomer and the D-isomer, have different properties. The L-isomer (poly-L-lactic acid [PLLA]) is hydrophobic and crystalline, with prolonged degradation time (up to several years), which makes it similar to nondegradable materials (in vivo behavior) and leads to late adverse reactions at the final stages of polymer degradation. The D-isomer is amorphous and less stable, properties that proved to be advantageous in building copolymers with the L-isomer.

However, adverse biological reactions to resorbable implants can present in varying levels of severity from mild fluid accumulation to discharging sinus formation to irreversible tissue damage. Although sometimes the reactions are mild enough to have no effect on the long-term outcome, in several studies, the reactions have been moderate to severe and have necessitated second surgeries. In most cases, the histologic picture is consistent. Polymeric debris is usually visible, both extracellularly and intracellularly, and osteolytic lesions are often found. Many factors affect the degradation of the polymer and the resulting reaction of the body to the polymer, including implant material, implant geometry, site of implantation, and method of sterilization. The results of the many published clinical trials show some common complications resulting from the widespread use of resorbable implants.[1,2]

More recently, several companies have commercially introduced new orthopedic implant devices in an effort to mitigate the problematic inflammatory local tissue response of bioabsorbable polymer implants by mixing powder of various mineral compositions into the bioabsorbable polymer compositions to create biocomposites. Some companies mixed in powder of tricalcium phosphate (Bioretec) or biphasic calcium phosphate (Arthrex), some mixed in hydroxyapatite (Takiron), some mixed in calcium sulfate, and some companies use mixtures of these powders (Stryker, Smith & Nephew). Such biocomposite implants usually incorporate 30% to 40% mineral content and the mineral content is entirely in the form of a fine powder, mixed into the polymer matrix. In all cases, the mineral powder is distributed homogeneously into the polymer composition. The mineral content in these implants can increase the brittleness of the implant because the mechanical strength of these implants derives primarily from the polymer and there is less polymer because of the mineral additives. This brittleness or weakness can lead to implant failure during insertion or subsequently in the postoperative period.

Because of the limited mechanical strength, biocomposite and bioabsorbable implants have been limited to specific clinical indications that do not require load-bearing levels of mechanical strength. The primary clinical indication for these biocomposite implants is in orthopedic sports medicine for soft tissue attachment (anterior cruciate ligament [ACL] interference screws, suture anchors, biotenodesis), in which cortical bone level strength is not required.

Even in soft tissue fixation, with regard to adverse inflammatory responses of biocomposites there remains a clinical problem. As Cox and colleagues[3] found, biocomposite ACL screws result in a high percentage of inflammatory reactions (cysts, edema). Furthermore, they do not encourage biointegration. As the article concludes, "Even though these newer-generation bioabsorbable screws were designed to promote osseous integration, no tunnel narrowing was noted."[3]

Mascarenhas and colleagues[4] found that, apart from these inflammatory problems, the current biocomposite screws also have mechanical problems: "The major findings of this study were prolonged knee effusion, increased femoral tunnel widening, and increased screw breakage associated with BIS [bioabsorbable interference screw] use."[4]

Thus, despite tremendous progress in biomaterials and bioabsorbable bone implants, surgeons and patients are still concerned with adverse tissue reactions caused by the degradation products of currently available bioresorbable orthopedic implant devices.[5] A strong clinical need remains for orthopedic implants that can provide mechanically secure fixation, integrate into the local tissue environment, and maintain an excellent in vivo safety and biocompatibility profile.

CURRENT THINKING ON RESORBABLE IMPLANTS

Recently, studies have begun on a new category of implant device technology that promises to bring mechanical and osteoconductive properties that are unprecedented in orthopedic biomaterials. These osteoconductive reinforced biocomposite implants are made from a reinforced biocomposite composed of two distinct components, each derived from a regulatory-approved family of biomaterials:

1. Reinforcing synthetic bone (mineral composition) fibers
2. Bioabsorbable polymer resin

The fibers provide superior mechanical properties to the implant and encourage bone ingrowth, whereas the polymer resin binds the fibers together into a cohesive element (**Fig. 1**). The reinforced mineral fibers are composed of a mineral blend that includes calcium, silica, magnesium, phosphorus, and several other minerals. This type of mineral blend is used in granule, putty, or paste form in several commercial (US Food and Drug Administration and CE [Conformité Européene] mark approved) synthetic bone filler products. These synthetic mineral fibers have been shown both in vitro and in vivo to be osteoconductive; ie, supporting bone growth and regeneration. The content of reinforcing mineral fibers within the reinforced biocomposite is more than 50%. This mineral content level is significantly greater than that of any commercially available biocomposite implant product. The reinforced biocomposite

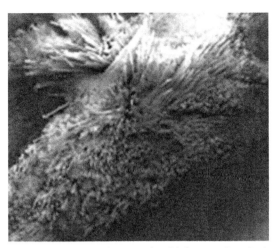

Fig. 1. Scanning electron microscope image of a biointegrative device. Reinforced bio-composite technology is unique in that the internal structure of each implant can be adapted to create the optimal biomechanical profile. This adaptation is achieved by designing and positioning thousands of mineral reinforcing fibers. Fibers are oriented to provide mechanical properties in different axes. (*Courtesy of* Ossio Ltd, Israel; with permission, rights reserved.)

implants undergo a progressive and balanced degradation process caused by the internal structure of the implants wherein the mineral fibers provide degradation channels that balance the polymer breakdown products. As such, these implants are not faced with the problematic inflammatory reaction seen in the current generation of biocomposite products (**Fig. 2**).

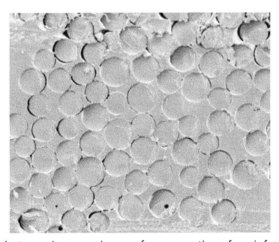

Fig. 2. Scanning electron microscope image of a cross section of a reinforced biocomposite implant in which the individual reinforcing fibers can be seen clearly. Each fiber is approximately 10 μm in diameter; about the same diameter as a human blood cell. Thousands, or even millions, of these tiny reinforcing fibers are combined to produce each implant. The biopolymer resin binds the fibers together such that the mechanical contributions of each of the fibers come together to create a biomechanically optimized implant. (*Courtesy of* Ossio Ltd, Israel; with permission, rights reserved.)

The mineral fiber content of reinforced biocomposites is integrated into bone. This process of biointegration is similar to the integration of synthetic bone filler products into the bone as the bone heals. The space that was filled with bone filler becomes filled with healthy bone. As the operated implantation site (bone fracture or osteotomy) gains strength during healing, the reinforced biocomposite implants gradually lose their strength, although they maintain their function for at least 12 weeks. Complete bone integration ultimately takes place, effectively eliminating the need for implant removal surgery.

Implant Structure

Reinforced biocomposite technology is unique in that the internal structure of each implant can be adapted to create the optimal biomechanical profile for that implant. This process is done by designing implants that are composed of thousands of mineral reinforcing fibers. The fibers can be aligned into fiber bundles that can be built into a variety of different structures. Fibers are oriented to provide mechanical properties in different mechanical axes. Within a single implant, there are thousands of distinct oriented fibers that provide the mechanical properties for that implant.

This process allows improved strength during insertion into bone because these implants do not bend or break easily during insertion. Because the previous bioabsorbable pins are much weaker than cortical bone, the insertion process into bone can result in high forces on the implant from the bone, which can cause it to break. This risk applies especially to implants of small diameter, such as pins or small screws.

Osteoconduction and Biointegration

The biopolymer content of the reinforced biocomposite material degrades by hydrolysis into alpha-hydroxy acids that are metabolized by the body. The mineral fiber content of the reinforced biocomposite is integrated and remodeled into bone.

Essentially, within the reinforced biocomposite material implants, two biological mechanisms occur concurrently: biopolymer bioresorption and mineral fiber biointegration. This hybrid material degradation mechanism enables that the absorption of the implants is pH balanced because the alpha-hydroxy acidic degradation products of the biopolymer are balanced by the alkaline degradation products of the mineral fibers. The hybrid degradation profile has great benefit in that it is balanced, progressive, and gradual. Interconnected pores are formed through the implant that allow fluid flow through the implant and potentially support physiologic regeneration of bone tissue in place of the implant as the implant degrades.

In previous bioabsorbable and biocomposite implants, the degradation profile was dominated by polymer bioresorption. Thus, there was suboptimal pH balance to mitigate the acidic degradation products of the polymer. There were no interconnected pores formed through the implant to allow gradual and progressive clearance of degradation products. The large biopolymer chains simply became weaker and weaker in place until, eventually, a burst release of acidic degradation products occurred. Because of the large size of the polymer chains, this burst release could occur even after several years and result in a severe local inflammatory reaction at the implant site years after the implant was introduced.

The reinforced biocomposite implants mechanistically avoid the burst release and inflammatory concerns that have been associated with previous bioabsorbable and biocomposite implants primarily because of a hybrid degradation profile that results in a balanced pH environment and interconnected pores that gradually and progressively allow fluid flow and clearance of degradation products from the local area of the implant. These factors result in a bioresorption profile in which the implant is safely and securely integrated into the local bone environment. The accumulation of biopolymer degradation products seen with previous bioabsorbable implants is avoided.

Mechanical Properties

The unique structural architecture of reinforced biocomposite technology provides mechanical benefit in several key ways:

Each reinforced biocomposite bone and soft tissue fixation implant is mechanically tested across multiple mechanical testing models in order to verify that the implant meets the specific biomechanical standards for the specified clinical indication. These tests can include bending force, shear force, tensile force, compressive force, torque resistance, and pull-out force. The reinforced biocomposite implant must be at least as strong as an existing orthopedic implant that has been previously approved for that clinical indication across all relevant mechanical measures.

Although each mechanical test is important in its own right, bending force can serve as a useful mechanical strength benchmark for many bone fixation implants because the bending axis is frequently the weak link in the mechanical performance of an implant. Therefore, it is crucial to assess whether an orthopedic implant's strength is sufficient to resist bending forces. When the bending modulus and strength that can be achieved with reinforced biocomposite is compared with those of bioabsorbable polymers (such as PLLA and self-reinforced PLLA) in the context of the mechanical properties of cortical bone, as shown in **Fig. 3**, it becomes clear that these polymers are far short of having the mechanical properties necessary to provide adequate fixation and reduction of bone. Only reinforced biocomposite has sufficient flexural modulus and strength to adequately fixate bone in load-bearing applications.

Animal Study Data

In order to show the osteoconductive properties of the reinforced biocomposite implant technology, an in-bone implantation study was performed.

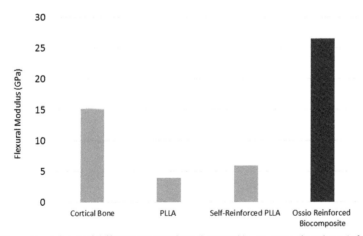

Fig. 3. Flexural modulus of differing materials and cortical bone. Note that the reinforced biocomposite material has better flexural modulus than previous materials used in absorbable implants and cortical bone. Ossio reinforced biocomposite implants are not yet commercially available.

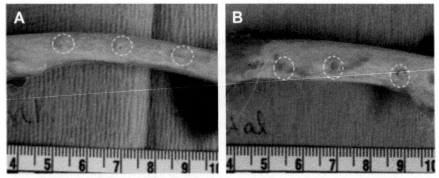

Fig. 4. A comparison of 26-week implantation sites of the reinforced biocomposite (*A*) versus a polymer implant (*B*). Note advanced integration of the biocomposite with surrounding bone, in comparison with the polymer implant. (*Courtesy of* Ossio Ltd, Israel, with permission, rights reserved).

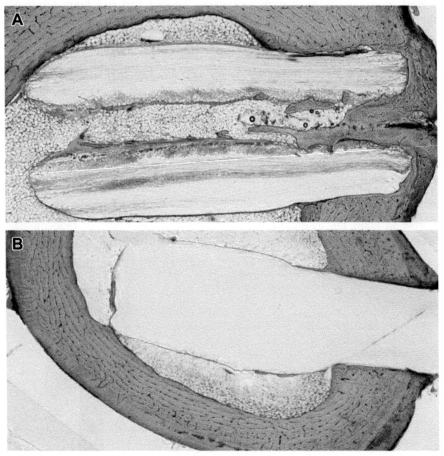

Fig. 5. Histology cross-section at 26 weeks in a rabbit femur (Stevenel's blue). A comparison between unicortical implantation sites of a reinforced biocomposite implant (*A*) and a polymer implant used for comparison (*B*). Note osseous ingrowth into the device lumen with incorporation of tissue within the mineral fibers (*A*), while no interaction is evident between the polymer implant and surrounding tissue (*B*). (*Courtesy of* Ossio Ltd, Israel, with permission, rights reserved).

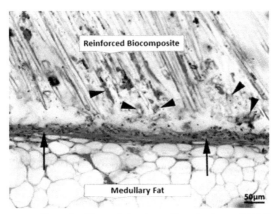

Fig. 6. Histology cross-section of a 13-week implantation site in a rabbit (hematoxylin-eosin). Reinforced biocomposite implanted in medullary canal. Arrows indicate a layer of connective tissue lining the edge of the implant; Arrowheads indicate ingrowth of mesenchymal tissue into wall of implant. (*Courtesy of* Ossio Ltd, Israel, with permission, rights reserved).

Reinforced biocomposite implants, 2 mm outer diameter, 1 mm inner diameter, 6 mm in length, were implanted unicortically into the mid-shaft of the right femur of rabbits. Absorbable polymer implants of the same outer diameter (without a lumen) were implanted in the same fashion into the contra-lateral femur for comparison. Femurs, implant sites and relevant lymph nodes were collected and evaluated at 4, 13, and 26 weeks to assess the potential for local irritation as well as to determine the bioresorption profile and osseous tissue ingrowth/integration into the implants.

Results

The bioresorption profile timelines differed greatly between the reinforced bio-composite and the polymer implants. The reinforced biocomposite implant showed evidence of substantial bioresorption of the polymer component through 26 weeks, as assessed by phagocytic activity. The absorbable polymer implant used for comparison showed only minimal evidence of fragmentation of the device at 26 weeks without evidence of an active or significant bioresorption process (**Figs. 4–7**). No evidence of safety concerns or adverse effects were documented throughout the study.

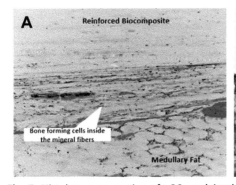
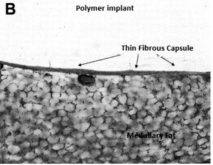

Fig. 7. Histology cross-section of a 26-week implantation site in a rabbit (hematoxylin-eosin). A comparison between unicortical implantation sites of a reinforced biocomposite implant (*A*) and polymer control (*B*). Bone forming cells can be seen between the mineral fibers of the reinforced biocomposite implant. (*Courtesy of* Ossio Ltd, Israel, with permission, rights reserved).

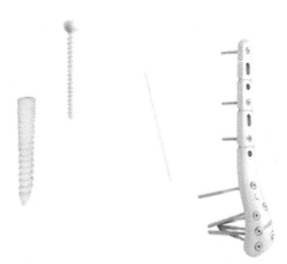

Fig. 8. Early product line design work showing potential uses as a pin, screw, interference screw, and multiple plate design options of biointegrative technology. Note that absorption can be set at differing time requirements and the screw, pin, or plate can be designed with differing regions of strength, thickness, and flex within each plate. (*Courtesy of* Ossio Ltd, Israel; with permission, rights reserved.)

SUMMARY

Advancement in orthopedics have been increasing rapidly. The most important advances have been in fixation. With time, metallic hardware will begin to be replaced by novel biomaterials that become one with the body. This progress will not only aid in the repair process it will allow permanent and improved reinforcement of the fixated region. Over time, it is expected that plates, screws, pins, interference screws, and even possibly joint replacements will incorporate into patients' bodies, negating the need for hardware removal and adding structure and stability to an iatrogenically weakened area (**Fig. 8**).

REFERENCES

1. Ambrose CG, Clanton TO. Bioabsorbable implants: review of clinical experience in orthopedic surgery. Ann Biomed Eng 2004;32(1):171–7.
2. Kontakis GM, Pagkalos JE, Tosounidis TI, et al. Bioabsorbable materials in orthopaedics. Acta Orthop Belg 2007;73:159–69.
3. Cox CL, Spindler KP, Leonard JP, et al. Do newer-generation bioabsorbable screws become incorporated into bone at two years after ACL reconstruction with patellar tendon graft? A cohort study. J Bone Joint Surg Am 2014;96:244–50.
4. Mascarenhas R, Saltzman BM, Sayegh ET, et al. Bioabsorbable versus metallic interference screws in anterior cruciate ligament reconstruction: a systematic review of overlapping meta-analyses. Arthroscopy 2015;31(3):561–8.
5. Konan S, Haddad FS. A clinical review of bioabsorbable interference screws and their adverse effects in anterior cruciate ligament reconstruction surgery. Knee 2009;16(1):6–13.

New Fixation Methods for the Treatment of the Diabetic Foot

Beaming, External Fixation, and Beyond

Roberto A. Brandão, DPM[a], Jeffrey S. Weber, DPM, AACFAS[b],
David Larson, DPM, AACFAS[c], Mark A. Prissel, DPM, AACFAS[a],
Patrick E. Bull, DO[a], Gregory C. Berlet, MD[a],
Christopher F. Hyer, DPM, MS[a],*

KEYWORDS

- Charcot neuroarthropathy • External fixation • Hindfoot reconstruction
- Midfoot beaming • Plate fixation • Superconstructs • Panfoot arthrodesis

KEY POINTS

- Multiple methods of fixation can be used in the successful reconstruction of the diabetic Charcot foot and ankle.
- New reconstruction-specific systems offer unique locking plates, beaming bolts, and screws that permit easy application with effective realignment and desired compression.
- Augmented external fixation and intramedullary nailing techniques are often used for complex hindfoot correction with successful limb salvage rates.
- Continual development of various fixation methods have helped to achieve long-term, successful outcomes.

INTRODUCTION

Charcot neuroarthropathy (CN) was originally described in 1703 by Sir William Musgrave secondary to complications of known venereal disease.[1,2] CN, later attributed to Jean Charcot, is an inflammatory arthropathy leading to joint destruction,

Disclosures: Drs G.C. Berlet and C.F. Hyer have disclosed the following conflicts: royalties, speaker's bureau, and consultant fees from Wright Medical Technology with products discussed in this article. Drs R.A. Brandão, D. Larson, and J.S. Weber have no disclosures. Dr P.E. Bull and Dr M.A. Prissel have no disclosures to note at this time.
^a Orthopedic Foot and Ankle Center, 300 Polaris Parkway, Westerville, OH 43082, USA;
^b Milwaukee Foot and Ankle Specialists, 3610 Michelle Witmer Memorial Drive, New Berlin, WI 53151, USA; ^c Integrated Orthopedics, 20940 North Tatum Boulevard, Suite B-290, Phoenix, Arizona 85050, USA
* Corresponding author.
E-mail address: ofacresearch@orthofootankle.com

Clin Podiatr Med Surg 35 (2018) 63–76
http://dx.doi.org/10.1016/j.cpm.2017.08.001
0891-8422/18/© 2017 Elsevier Inc. All rights reserved.

instability, and deformity of the foot and ankle.[1,3] In 1936, William Riley Jordon reported on the high association of CN with diabetes mellitus (DM) and recognized DM as the primary cause of distal peripheral neuropathy.[1,2] Patients with neuropathic fracture dislocations with subsequent midfoot or hindfoot deformities are at increased risk for soft tissue ulcerations, osteomyelitis, major lower extremity amputation, and a reduced quality of life.[1,4] The goals of both nonoperative and operative management are to reduce rates of minor and major amputations through creation of a stable, plantigrade, and ulceration-free foot.[5–7]

Globally, more than 350 million people are affected with diabetes with estimates nearing 600 million by 2035.[8,9] The Centers for Disease Control and Prevention estimated that approximately 9.3% of Americans are living with DM, and nearly 28% are unaware of their diagnosis.[2,10] With the reported incidence of CN between 0.1 and 5% of those with diabetic neuropathy, treatment of its many complications continues to evolve in the medical and surgical realms of medicine.[5,11] This continued interest has fostered progressive research and new technological advancements leading to a shift toward amputation reduction via stronger emphasis on surgical management for CN ulceration. The surgical management of the CN foot and ankle requires robust fixation strategies to provide consistent long-term stability and deformity reduction. These fixation methods are the focus of this article (**Fig. 1**).

RECONSTRUCTION TRENDS AND PRINCIPLES

When nonsurgical treatment of the CN foot has failed secondary to persistent deformity, progression to a nonbraceable deformity, or limb-threatening ulceration,

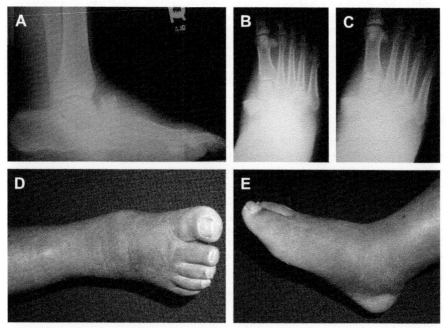

Fig. 1. (*A–C*) Lateral, anteroposterior, and oblique plain film radiographs of a patient with a midfoot CN deformity with a dorsally and medially dislocated navicular without talonavicular joint instability. (*D, E*) Clinical photographs demonstrate increased redness and pedal edema, consistent with physical examination findings of CN.

surgical intervention is indicated. New fixation techniques have changed the way surgeons evaluate and treat complex deformities along with continued expansion on recently updated treatment principles. The authors think that the traditional principles of plate-screw fixation and limited resection have a very small role in the modern management of diabetic foot and ankle CN. In 2009, Sammarco[12] presented the concept of *superconstructs* when discussing the advent of plantar plating, axial loading screws, and locking plate technology. The superconstructs surgical treatment principles represent the more modern understanding of CN and include the following:

- Extension of surgical fusion beyond the zone of injury (Charcot) to include unaffected joints and therefore improving construct stability.
- The utilization of the strongest device possible that does not compromise soft tissue coverage.
- Bone resection as needed to reduce the deformity by means of shortening, allowing for reduced tension of the soft tissues.
- Application of devices in a position of maximal mechanical advantage.

Building upon the supercontruct concept, Mallory and colleagues[13] presented a "panfoot arthrodesis" approach to CN fixation in 2015. The investigators presented a small case series of 9 patients with CN midfoot deformity who underwent surgical fixation based on previously described anatomic classification.[14] Reduction in Meary's angle, dorsal displacement, and talar declination were observed postoperatively. No reported midfoot hardware failure occurred during the 12-month follow-up period. The aims of the technique included the following:

- Ankle and hindfoot equinus must be addressed before midfoot deformity correction.
- Fixation constructs need not extend across the tibiotalar joint in isolated Lisfranc joint deformities.
- More proximal deformity (ie, Chopart) correction should incorporate a tibiotalar arthrodesis.
- Subtalar joint arthrodesis is used in all cases of midfoot collapse regardless of collapse location or ankle CN involvement.

Although the use of internal fixation has evolved, surgical management of CN can be complicated by the presence of a plantar foot ulceration and osteomyelitis. Eradication of infection remains a steadfast principle of the CN reconstruction management. At times, this would contraindicate internal fixation and necessitate the need for external stabilization. Wukich and colleagues[15] recently reviewed 245 patients with CN over a 10-year period. The investigators found that 164 patients had active wounds, with most having deep soft tissue or bone infection. Surgical options included irrigation and debridement, exostectomy, staged reconstruction, and primary amputation. Patients with ulceration were less likely to be treated with only internal fixation; conversely, external fixation was 16 times more likely to be used without any combination of internal fixation. Infection management is an integral part of CN management that can be aided by the advent of new technology.

With the advent of new Charcot reconstruction-specific fixation systems for the foot and ankle, surgeons have the ability to offer enhanced long-term midfoot or hindfoot stability to the deformed Charcot foot. This article seeks to outline these new technologies in CN reconstruction, including plating constructs with locking screws, axial beaming with solid bolts and screws, retrograde hindfoot intramedullary nailing (IMN), in addition to the uses of external fixation (**Fig. 2**).

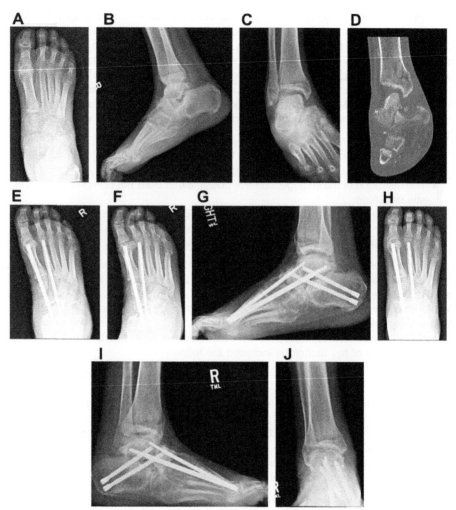

Fig. 2. (*A–D*) Preoperative anteroposterior, lateral, and oblique foot and ankle plain film radiographs and computed tomographic evaluation of a complete subtalar joint dislocation in a type 2 diabetic male with peripheral neuropathy. Noted varus deformity of the midfoot is seen. (*E–G*) Postoperative images with medial column arthrodesis using bolt fixation and concomitant subtalar joint arthrodesis with fully threaded screws. (*H–J*) Follow-up images of the same patient demonstrate the application of the superconstructs for CN deformity reduction.

MIDFOOT
Midfoot Locking Screw and Plate Fixation

The use of internal fixation for midfoot Charcot deformity correction has been widely reported with good outcomes.[2,16,17] The midtarsal joints are commonly affected in CN. Stabilizing these joints requires unique fixation strategies secondary to ongoing and recurrent instability, which lead to severe fracture fragmentation and collapse of the pedal architecture.[14,18] One method of midfoot fixation for the Charcot foot that has been used is plantar plating. The theory behind this form of fixation lends to the inherent stability of the plate on the tension side of the deforming forces exerted on the midfoot during weight-bearing. The extensive dissection required for this technique has led to other methods of fixation becoming more of the mainstay for the CN foot. One such method is the extended medial column plating system, which maximizes construct stability while minimizing soft tissue dissection.[12,19,20] Traditional nonlocking fixation for joint arthrodesis or buttressing has evolved into stronger and more stable joint-specific contoured reconstruction locking systems. Extended medial column arthrodesis through medial plating has been advocated by several investigators to restore alignment, enhancing construct stability and promoting earlier postoperative functional recovery in midfoot reconstruction.[18–21]

Acceptance and indoctrination of the superconstructs principles have led to the abandonment of conventional nonlocking plate fixation for midfoot CN. Biomechanically, locking plate constructs have shown superiority in load to failure rates when compared with traditional plating methods.[22] Whether for periarticular fracture reduction or buttressing for angular deformity maintenance, locking plates can provide enhanced stability in both primary and revision cases. Unlike nonlocking systems, locking plate constructs can provide stability in osteopenic bone created by the destructive CN process. Another added benefit of modern locking plate technology is variable angle or polyaxial screws. Recent studies have found that polyaxial screw application in a locking plate can enhance stability and allow for more varied application than uniaxial screw fixation.[21,23] Polyaxial plating systems can be particularly advantageous in midfoot deformity correction with highly comminuted fracture patterns where solid screw purchase may be dependent on angulation into a specific fixation point.

Charcot indicated–specific plates such as the SALVATION 3Di Plating System (Wright Medical Technology, Inc, Arlington, TN, USA) can be used for extended medial column arthrodesis through the talonavicular, naviculocuneiform, and 1st tarsometatarsal joints as previously described.[18] The bridging and reconstruction plates allow for nonlocking and locking screws in both the applications for extended medial column arthrodesis. To reduce the need for plantar dissection, each plate is anatomically designed for medial column application with specified laterality in 3 sizes. The plate also contains a compression slot for a nonlocking screw after proximal fixation is achieved. The bridging plates offer the most screw holes for maximum fixation while allowing for a contoured fit along the medial column. Because of the varied fixation options within this plate, bone graft can be used when having multiple points to secure the plate around the grafting site. The reconstruction plate can allow for proximal midfoot fixation with 2 compression slots for midfoot arthrodesis in a similar fashion to the bridging plate. Both plates have a low profile footprint, which allow for increased soft tissue coverage, which can be a complicating factor in CN reconstruction management. The screws can be inserted poly-axially in a nonlocking and locking manner with variable degree of angulation to aid in purchasing tenuous bone. Although midfoot plating offers added strength due to its multiple fixation points, other methods of correction may be used for CN reconstruction and have their own inherent advantages over plating (**Fig. 3**).

Midfoot Beaming

As previously noted, diabetes is the most common cause of the peripheral neuropathy contributing to the development of foot and ankle CN. Wound healing in diabetic patients can be impaired by reduced macrophagic activity, reduced angiogenesis causing delayed healing, and high risk for infection.[24] Given the need for appropriate soft tissue management, one inherent disadvantage of midfoot plating systems,

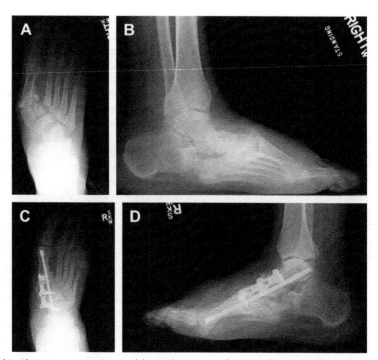

Fig. 3. (*A, B*) Anteroposterior and lateral images of a significant midfoot CN deformity with subluxation of the talonavicular and naviculocuneiform joint with dislocation of the 1st tarsometatarsal joint. Increased talar declination and dorsal dislocation of the 1st metatarsal is noted on the lateral view. Hypertrophic fracture fragmentation, and intermetatarsal and cuneiform diastasis are evident on the anteroposterior view. (*C, D*) Postoperative midfoot Charcot deformity reconstruction with medial extended fusion plating with concurrent medial beam fixation. (*Courtesy of* Carroll Jones MD, Charlotte, NC.)

locking or nonlocking, is the soft tissue dissection required for plate application. Concurrently, the soft tissue envelope may not be amenable to plating secondary to reduced skin pliability or edema. Recently, researchers have proposed intramedullary axial screw or bolt fixation, or "beaming," as a means to surgically restore medial and lateral column alignment with minimal dissection.[17,25–30] Biomechanically, beaming screws and bolts are capable of resisting axial loading forces across the midtarsal joints. Insertion of the beams along the medial column has been described from the 1st metatarsal head distally, and through the tarsometatarsal, naviculocuneiform, and talonavicular joint for stability. Placement of the lateral column beam can be completed from the 4th or 5th metatarsal in a similar retrograde fashion across the calcaneocuboid joint. Recently, Peterson and Hyer[31] described a percutaneous posterolateral insertion technique using a cadaveric model. Appropriate alignment was achieved, but the sural nerve was found to be at risk during insertion. Sural nerve damage may be a small limiting factor given the neuropathic nature of CN patients. More prospective research is needed to elucidate success rates of this technique in vivo.

In 2011, Grant and colleagues[27] reported on 71 Charcot foot reconstructions using medial and lateral beaming with 6.5-mm partially threaded screws. The investigators noted significant overall radiographic improvement in alignment of both the medial and the lateral columns using a standard approach for beaming. When using a 6.5-mm partially threaded cannulated screw, the researchers noted failure of the screw at the "run out" in 4 patients. Previous reports, including works by Sammarco and colleagues[17] and Assal and Stern,[26] noted screw breakage in 36.4% and 26.7% of their study patients, respectively. Assal and Stern[26] surgically corrected 15 patients using an 8-mm diameter by 150-mm length screw for "stronger fixation," in addition to lateral column beaming and dorsal midfoot plate fixation. Four nonunions occurred along the medial column, with only one patient losing significant clinical and radiographic reduction. Lamm and colleagues[32] proposed that the increased screw diameter and added fixation points of this system contributed to successful and maintained realignment arthrodesis.[27,32] In 2012, Lamm and colleagues[32] discussed the advantages of intramedullary foot fixation (IMFF) for midfoot CN correction.[32] The study concluded that IMFF offered appropriate anatomic alignment, rigid fixation, preservation of foot length, and adherence to superconstruct principles by fixating beyond the immediate zone of injury. They used 7.0-/8.0-mm cannulated fully threaded screws for multiple points of the fixation through both central and lateral columns but did not report on complications. The SALVATION Fusion Beam (Wright Medical Technology, Inc, Arlington, TN, USA) 7.0-mm cannulated screws are made from type II anodized titanium alloy and are available in both partial and fully threaded patterns. Through use of a cannulated technique, the medial and lateral column screw fixation systems allow for easy application. Although the relative ease of application and minimal soft tissue compromise are promising, surgeons must be aware of hardware complications that can occur and augment fixation as needed for enhanced structural support.

Although screws have shown success in achieving and supporting realignment, recent advancements in beaming hardware seek to further enhance stability of medial column constructs. New indication-specific medial column bolts (MCB) are designed to withstand the compressive and tensile forces experienced within the intramedullary canal.[29] In 2013, Cullen and colleagues[29] reported on a small series of 4 patients using a 6.5-mm solid Midfoot Fusion Bolt (Synthes, Solothurn, Switzerland) for medial column arthrodesis. Concurrent lateral column stabilization was achieved with 7.3-mm cannulated screws placed antegrade from the calcaneus to the cuboid. All deformity correction was maintained at 12 months with one bolt migration noted, and no major complications reported. Similarly, Wiewiorski and colleagues[28] performed MCB using identical hardware with an average 27-month follow-up and concluded that alignment was maintained in 7 of 8 patients with no recurrent ulcerations. A recent meta-analysis of MCB for CN reconstruction in 191 patients resulted in improvement of deformity, and complications were reduced if additional fixation was used. The SALVATION Fusion Bolts (Wright Medical Technology, Inc, Arlington, TN, USA) are solid compression screws that are available in 5.0-mm and 6.5-mm sizes. Given their smaller intramedullary canal diameters, narrower screw options are available for beaming of the middle and lateral columns. The larger bolts are ideal for medial longitudinal beaming from the 1st metatarsal head into the talus with the ability to compress through all midfoot joints (**Fig. 4**).

INTRAMEDULLARY NAIL FIXATION

Surgical management of the hindfoot and ankle CN is another challenge due to gross instability and potential for limb-threatening infection secondary to ulceration. A recent systematic review by Schneekloth and colleagues[2] reported on 860 Charcot surgeries from 2006 to 2014; the most common area of surgical intervention was the hindfoot (41.6%) and ankle (38.4%), respectively. One of the most common procedures performed on the hindfoot and ankle was a tibiotalocalcaneal (TTC) arthrodesis, used

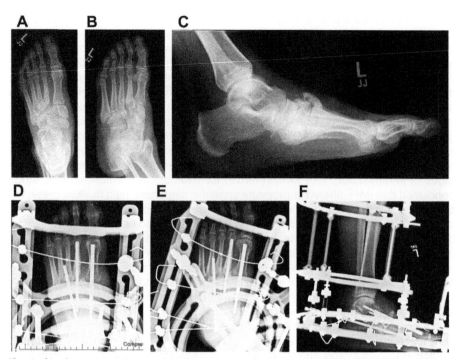

Fig. 4. (*A–C*) Anteroposterior, oblique, and lateral preoperative plain film radiographs of the Lisfranc-level CN deformity with dorsal fracture subluxation and transverse plane diastasis. (*D–F*) Example of midfoot bolt fixation of a medial column along with screw fixation of the lateral column in the setting of concomitant external fixation application for a reconstruction. Note the posterior orientated insertion of the lateral column screw (*E, F*).

in 70 of the 860 (19.8%) surgeries with no specific fixation type discussed. This "increasing trend" of TTC arthrodesis can be accomplished with several different forms of fixation, including cannulated or solid screw fixation, lateral humeral locking plates, external fixation, and retrograde IMN.[2,6,33–35] One emerging fixation method, retrograde IMN, can offer surgeons a stable, loading-sharing fixation with the ability to resist torsional forces.[11,15] As the need continues to evolve for a consistent and reproducible means of gross deformity correction in hindfoot and ankle CN, the use of IMN can create a solid or stable fibrous union amenable to brace ambulation, limb salvage, and reduced complications.[11]

Intramedullary nail fixation has been increasingly cited in the literature for CN hindfoot deformity correction.[7,15,33] DeVries and colleagues[33] discussed the use of retrograde IMN fixation for the stabilization of CN ankle deformities in 52 patients with 7 of the patients also receiving combined external fixation application. The investigators noted a 77.8% limb salvage rate for the IMN group over a mean follow-up period of 101 weeks. In 2015, Wukich and colleagues[7] reported on 117 patients, 61 with DM and 56 without, undergoing TTC arthrodesis for various indications. A subset of the study included 51 patients being treated for CN. They noted a limb salvage rate of 95.7% overall for both DM and non-DM groups. In a smaller study, Siebachmeyer and colleagues[36] presented 20 patients with severe deformity of the hindfoot in the setting of CN. Fifteen patients had concurrent ulcerations at the time of correction, and 7 were treated with adjunctive midfoot beaming and plate fixation as needed. The overall limb salvage rate was 100%, and 80% of patients had healed ulcerations by the end of the mean 26-month follow-up period. Recently, Ettinger and colleagues[37] performed surgical treatment on 58 CN patients with ankle joint involvement. The investigators used intramedullary nail technique and achieved 100% successful arthrodesis in 38 patients at a mean follow-up period of 31.3 months.

The increased use of IMN fixation for CN hindfoot and ankle reconstruction has fostered continued innovation of retrograde hindfoot arthrodesis systems. Mann and colleagues[38] demonstrated that a retrograde IMN with a posterior-to-anterior interlocking screw through the calcaneus provided increased stabilization compared with conventional transverse screw fixation.[38] In response to this research, implant companies have developed retrograde hindfoot nailing systems intended specifically for CN hindfoot reconstruction. The Valor Hindfoot Fusion Nail (Wright Medical Technology, Inc, Arlington, TN, USA), T2 Ankle Arthrodesis Nail (Stryker, Mahwah, NJ, USA), and Expert Hindfoot Arthrodesis Nail (HAN; Depuy Synthes, Warsaw, IN, USA) are 3 such systems. Each system offers unique angulation, the ability to create dynamization with dynamic screw placement and compression for primary fusion. The Expert HAN has a distinctive 12° distal lateral bend to the nail with a spiral blade inserted within the calcaneus perpendicular to the long axis of the nail secured by fixed-angle locking end cap. The HAN has been noted to offer good stability in osteoporotic and nonosteoporotic bone in hindfoot arthrodesis.[39] The T2 Ankle Arthrodesis Nail has been used for CN hindfoot arthrodesis and deformity correction by Wukich and colleagues[7] in their previously mentioned study. The T2 offers a 5° valgus bend for soft tissue and neurovascular protection with a 5.0-mm interlocking posterior-to-anterior calcaneal locking screw. The system also has an internal "compression screw" intended for advancing compression across the tibiotalar joint and an external compression through the "apposition handle" across the talocalcaneal joint. The Valor Hindfoot Fusion Nail varies from the aforementioned systems because it uses a straight, nonangulation design for hindfoot arthrodesis. This system also allows for tibiotalar and talocalcaneal compression, although it is done all internally by the "internal compression screw." In addition, it has the ability to perform conjunctive subtalar joint stabilization through the nail device with the "subtalar screw." IMN has become a more established treatment form of hindfoot CN reconstruction, and hardware advances cater to the unique anatomy and fixation needs for successful management (**Fig. 5**).

EXTERNAL FIXATION

External fixation in conjunction with internal fixation has gained popularity in the surgical management of complex midfoot and hindfoot CN deformities. External fixation can be used in both static and dynamic forms to stabilize deformity and to protect soft tissues. The application of external fixation to the foot and ankle is useful for wound offloading, for wound stabilization in plastics reconstruction, and as a multipart staging for acute and chronic deformities related to CN.[40,41] Poor bone quality, ulceration, and a compromised soft tissue envelope do not preclude the use of external fixation, making it a viable option for midfoot or hindfoot stabilization when internal fixation is contraindicated. Its percutaneous application technique makes it the perfect stabilization option in the presence of active infection or osteomyelitis in a staged manner where internal fixation would be contraindicated.[15]

Single surgery or staged surgical management of CN is an excellent use for external circular-frame fixation when osteomyelitis or ulceration is present. Pinzur and colleagues[6] described a single-stage correction with static circular ring external fixation in patients with CN and concurrent osteomyelitis. They reported a 95.7% limb salvage rate at 1- year follow-up.[6] In addition, hindfoot arthrodesis with external

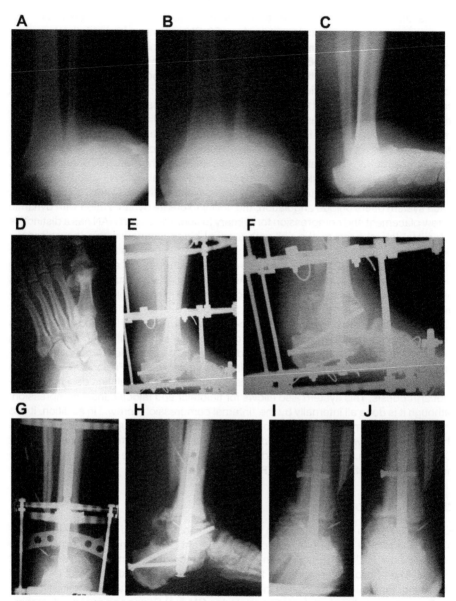

Fig. 5. (*A–D*) Plain film images demonstrate severe hindfoot Charcot deformity with dislocation of the hindfoot at the level of the ankle joint. (*E–J*) The deformity was reduced, and the alignment was maintained using intramedullary nail fixation as a means of primary internal stabilization and femoral head allograft implantation. In addition, the graft and subtalar joint were further stabilized with screw fixation through the inferior aspect of the nail. External fixation was also applied as a secondary means of fixation.

fixation in the presence of infection has been described by Fabrin and colleagues[42] with a successful limb salvage rate of 92%. Management of active or consolidated CN with a staged protocol using external fixation for reduction correction, soft tissue maintenance, and ulcer management has been more commonly reported.[34,43]

Monaco and colleagues[43] presented a case of a lateral subtalar joint dislocation in a neuropathic insulin-controlled diabetic man with clinical warmth, edema, impending ulceration, and previous MRI (performed before referral) consistent with CN. The investigators staged the reconstruction using a multiplanar external fixator (The Distraction Osteogenesis Ring System, Depuy Synthes, Warsaw, IN, USA) for gross hindfoot realignment with subsequent pantalar arthrodesis 10 weeks after the index procedure. The patient remained ulcer free with a plantigrade foot at 1-year follow-up. Combined internal and external fixation, as recently described by Hegewald and colleagues,[34] whom performed 22 CN reconstructions of both the midfoot (16) and hindfoot (6) using a static Ilizarov external fixator in addition to internal medial column and TTC arthrodesis, demonstrated successful limb salvage rates (90.91%) over a mean follow-up period of 58 weeks.

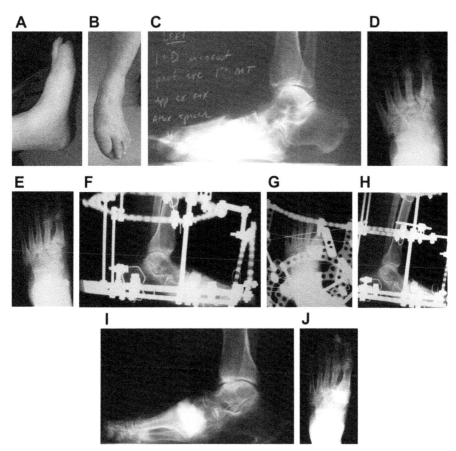

Fig. 6. (*A–E*) Preoperative clinical and radiographic images of midfoot Charcot collapse rocker bottom deformity. Notable midfoot collapse with subsequent fracture of the 1st metatarsal and midfoot fragmentation. Plantar prominence is seen on the lateral image, now with the presence of a plantar midfoot ulceration. (*F–H*) The use of external fixation here reduced the deformity with additional use of antibiotic spacer and plantar exostectomy for prominence resection. (*I, J*) Postoperative images after the external fixator was removed demonstrate a reduced deformity with no plantar prominence.

Lamm and colleagues[44] described a percutaneous technique using the Taylor Spatial Frame (Smith & Nephew, Memphis, TN, USA) for gradual CN deformity correction. They describe a 2-stage approach with initial osseous realignment followed by application of gradual external fixation correction in 11 feet. The construct was finalized with medial column beaming. The SALVATION External Fixation System (Wright Medical Technology, Inc, Arlington, TN, USA) circular multiplanar frame is indicated for arthrodesis, hindfoot stabilization, offloading, and traumatic fracture management. As with many external fixation systems, this system can be used in conjunction with internal fixation as deemed appropriate. The preassembled ring constructs increase intraoperative efficiency. To consistently ensure optimal leg position within the external fixator, the system offers easily applied leg positioners that can be temporarily attached to the frame. The versatile nature of the open slotted ring design allows for faster and less cumbersome attachment to half-pins and wires. Wire guides are available for proper placement of the wire to reduce wire bending during insertion. An additional unique feature of the SALVATION (Wright Medical Technology, Inc, Arlington, TN, USA) system is a rocker plate, which can be used for wound offloading or frame protection weight-bearing if indicated (**Fig. 6**).

SUMMARY

Reconstruction of the foot and ankle secondary to CN collapse is a complicated and technically challenging endeavor. New fixation techniques respecting superconstructs principles and the extended arthrodesis theories have established a paradigm shift in complex CN deformity management. Charcot-specific reconstruction systems provide surgeons with a novel approach to addressing complex CN surgical problem limb salvage.

REFERENCES

1. Wukich DK, Sung W. Charcot arthropathy of the foot and ankle: modern concepts and management review. J Diabet Complications 2009;23(6):409–26.
2. Schneekloth BJ, Lowery NJ, Wukich DK. Charcot neuroarthropathy in patients with diabetes: an updated systematic review of surgical management. J Foot Ankle Surg 2016;55(3):586–90.
3. Gupta R. A short history of neuropathic arthropathy. Clin Orthop Relat Res 1993;(296):43–9.
4. Raspovic KM, Wukich DK. Self-reported quality of life in patients with diabetes: a comparison of patients with and without Charcot neuroarthropathy. Foot Ankle Int 2014;35(3):195–200.
5. La Fontaine J, Lavery L, Jude E. Current concepts of Charcot foot in diabetic patients. Foot (Edinb) 2016;26:7–14.
6. Pinzur MS, Gil J, Belmares J. Treatment of osteomyelitis in Charcot foot with single-stage resection of infection, correction of deformity, and maintenance with ring fixation. Foot Ankle Int 2012;33(12):1069–74.
7. Wukich DK, Mallory BR, Suder NC, et al. Tibiotalocalcaneal arthrodesis using retrograde intramedullary nail fixation: comparison of patients with and without diabetes mellitus. J Foot Ankle Surg 2015;54(5):876–82.
8. Seuring T, Archangelidi O, Suhrcke M. The economic costs of type 2 diabetes: a global systematic review. Pharmacoeconomics 2015;33(8):811–31.
9. International Diabetes Federation. IDF diabetes atlas. In: Guariguata L, Nolan T, Beagley J, et al, editors. 6th edition. Brussels, Belgium: International Diabetes Federation; 2013. p. 12–3. Available at: www.idf.org/diabetesatlas.

10. Centers for Disease Control and Prevention. National diabetes statistics report: estimates of diabetes and its burden in the United States. Atlanta (GA): U.S. Department of Health and Human Services; 2014.

11. Ogut T, Yontar NS. Surgical treatment options for the diabetic Charcot hindfoot and ankle deformity. Clin Podiatr Med Surg 2017;34(1):53–67.

12. Sammarco VJ. Superconstructs in the treatment of Charcot foot deformity: plantar plating, locked plating, and axial screw fixation. Foot Ankle Clin 2009;14(3): 393–407.

13. Mallory D, Dikis A, Highlander P, et al. Panfoot Arthrodesis: A Novel Technique for Management of Challenging Midfoot Charcot Deformity. American College of Foot and Ankle Surgeons Annual Scientific Meeting. Phoenix (AZ), February 19–22, 2015.

14. Brodsky JW, Rouse AM. Exostectomy for symptomatic bony prominences in diabetic Charcot feet. Clin Orthop Relat Res 1993;(296):21–6.

15. Wukich DK, Raspovic KM, Hobizal KB, et al. Surgical management of Charcot neuroarthropathy of the ankle and hindfoot in patients with diabetes. Diabetes Metab Res Rev 2016;32(Suppl 1):292–6.

16. Dayton P, Feilmeier M, Thompson M, et al. Comparison of complications for internal and external fixation for Charcot reconstruction: a systematic review. J Foot Ankle Surg 2015;54(6):1072–5.

17. Sammarco VJ, Sammarco GJ, Walker EW Jr, et al. Midtarsal arthrodesis in the treatment of Charcot midfoot arthropathy. J Bone Joint Surg Am 2009;91(1): 80–91.

18. Capobianco CM, Stapleton JJ, Zgonis T. The role of an extended medial column arthrodesis for Charcot midfoot neuroarthropathy. Diabet Foot Ankle 2010;1. http://dx.doi.org/10.3402/dfa.v1i0.5282.

19. Garchar D, DiDomenico LA, Klaue K. Reconstruction of Lisfranc joint dislocations secondary to Charcot neuroarthropathy using a plantar plate. J Foot Ankle Surg 2013;52(3):295–7.

20. Marks RM, Parks BG, Schon LC. Midfoot fusion technique for neuroarthropathic feet: biomechanical analysis and rationale. Foot Ankle Int 1998;19(8):507–10.

21. Cullen AB, Curtiss S, Lee MA. Biomechanical comparison of polyaxial and uniaxial locking plate fixation in a proximal tibial gap model. J Orthop Trauma 2009; 23(7):507–13.

22. Jastifer JR. Topical review: locking plate technology in foot and ankle surgery. Foot Ankle Int 2014;35(5):512–8.

23. Fidler CM, Prissel MA, Hyer CF. Locking plates: what have we learned? Podiatry Today 2015;28(9).

24. Brem H, Tomic-Canic M. Cellular and molecular basis of wound healing in diabetes. J Clin Invest 2007;117(5):1219–22.

25. Ahluwalia RS, O'dak S, Reichert IL, et al. The medial column fusion bolt. Foot Ankle Orthop 2016;1(1). 2473011416S2473000302.

26. Assal M, Stern R. Realignment and extended fusion with use of a medial column screw for midfoot deformities secondary to diabetic neuropathy. J Bone Joint Surg Am 2009;91(4):812–20.

27. Grant WP, Garcia-Lavin S, Sabo R. Beaming the columns for Charcot diabetic foot reconstruction: a retrospective analysis. J Foot Ankle Surg 2011;50(2):182–9.

28. Wiewiorski M, Yasui T, Miska M, et al. Solid bolt fixation of the medial column in Charcot midfoot arthropathy. J Foot Ankle Surg 2013;52(1):88–94.

29. Cullen BD, Weinraub GM, Van Gompel G. Early results with use of the midfoot fusion bolt in Charcot arthropathy. J Foot Ankle Surg 2013;52(2):235–8.

30. Fidler C, Watson BC, Reb CW, et al. Beaming in Charcot arthropathy-intramedullary fixation for complicated reconstructions: a cadaveric study. J Foot Ankle Surg 2017;56(4):802–4.

31. Peterson KS, Hyer CF. Posterior approach for medial column beam screw in midfoot Charcot reconstruction: technique and structures at risk. J Foot Ankle Surg 2015;54(3):433–6.

32. Lamm BM, Siddiqui NA, Nair AK, et al. Intramedullary foot fixation for midfoot Charcot neuroarthropathy. J Foot Ankle Surg 2012;51(4):531–6.

33. DeVries JG, Berlet GC, Hyer CF. A retrospective comparative analysis of Charcot ankle stabilization using an intramedullary rod with or without application of circular external fixator–utilization of the Retrograde Arthrodesis Intramedullary Nail database. J Foot Ankle Surg 2012;51(4):420–5.

34. Hegewald KW, Wilder ML, Chappell TM, et al. Combined internal and external fixation for diabetic Charcot reconstruction: a retrospective case series. J Foot Ankle Surg 2016;55(3):619–27.

35. Lee DJ, Schaffer J, Chen T, et al. Internal versus external fixation of Charcot midfoot deformity realignment. Orthopedics 2016;39(4):e595–601.

36. Siebachmeyer M, Boddu K, Bilal A, et al. Outcome of one-stage correction of deformities of the ankle and hindfoot and fusion in Charcot neuroarthropathy using a retrograde intramedullary hindfoot arthrodesis nail. Bone Joint J 2015;97B(1):76–82.

37. Ettinger S, Plaass C, Claassen L, et al. Surgical management of Charcot deformity for the foot and ankle-radiologic outcome after internal/external fixation. J Foot Ankle Surg 2016;55(3):522–8.

38. Mann MR, Parks BG, Pak SS, et al. Tibiotalocalcaneal arthrodesis: a biomechanical analysis of the rotational stability of the Biomet Ankle Arthrodesis Nail. Foot Ankle Int 2001;22(9):731–3.

39. Richter M, Evers J, Waehnert D, et al. Biomechanical comparison of stability of tibiotalocalcaneal arthrodesis with two different intramedullary retrograde nails. Foot Ankle Surg 2014;20(1):14–9.

40. Frykberg RG, Bevilacqua NJ, Habershaw G. Surgical off-loading of the diabetic foot. J Vasc Surg 2010;52(3 Suppl):44S–58S.

41. Ramanujam CL, Zgonis T. An overview of internal and external fixation methods for the diabetic Charcot foot and ankle. Clin Podiatr Med Surg 2017;34(1):25–31.

42. Fabrin J, Larsen K, Holstein P. Arthrodesis with external fixation in the unstable or misaligned Charcot ankle in patients with diabetes mellitus. J Low Extrem Wounds 2007;6:102–7.

43. Monaco S, Burns P, Toth A. Staged reconstruction for acute Charcot's subtalar joint dislocationa case report. J Am Podiatr Med Assoc 2016;106(6):445–8.

44. Lamm BM, Gottlieb HD, Paley D. A two-stage percutaneous approach to Charcot diabetic foot reconstruction. J Foot Ankle Surg 2010;49(6):517–22.

Next-Generation, Minimal-Resection, Fixed-Bearing Total Ankle Replacement
Indications and Outcomes

Justin Tsai, MS, MD[a], David I. Pedowitz, MS, MD[b],*

KEYWORDS

- Arthroplasty • Fixed • Minimal • Modern • Ankle

KEY POINTS

- Total ankle arthroplasty is being performed more frequently in recent years, and the increase in use has been accompanied by innovative changes in implant design.
- Features of 1 new implant include minimal bone resection, condylar shape of the talar component, anatomic contouring of the tibial component to maximize surface area and prevent malleolar impingement, and the ability to adjust for subluxation in the sagittal plane using anteriorly or posteriorly biased polyethylene inserts.
- Some of these features are shared among many of the newer available implants, indicating a general consensus in the foot and ankle community on what is important in arthroplasty design. Further studies need to be done to document intermediate and long-term outcomes.

INTRODUCTION

Arthritis is a debilitating disease that causes pain and dysfunction, affecting the ability of those affected to carry out activities of daily living. It is currently thought to disable about 10% of people older than 60-years-old and compromise the quality of life of more than 20 million Americans.[1] Although the impact of endstage hip and knee arthritis on quality of life is well-documented,[2,3] the data on ankle arthritis have been scarce until more recently. A recent study found that mental and physical disabilities were comparable between patients with endstage ankle and hip arthrosis.[4] This, combined with the fact that ankle arthritis is less common, may be a reason why

The authors have nothing to disclose.
a Department of Orthopaedic Surgery, SUNY Downstate College of Medicine, 450 Clarkson Avenue, Brooklyn, NY 11203, USA; b The Rothman Institute, 925 Chestnut Street, Philadelphia, PA 19107, USA
* Corresponding author.
E-mail address: David.Pedowitz@rothmaninstitute.com

Clin Podiatr Med Surg 35 (2018) 77–83
http://dx.doi.org/10.1016/j.cpm.2017.08.005
0891-8422/18/© 2017 Elsevier Inc. All rights reserved.

technical and clinical advancements in total ankle arthroplasty have lagged behind those seen in hip and knee arthroplasty.

Ankle arthrodesis has traditionally been the gold standard for endstage tibiotalar arthritis, but recent studies comparing arthroplasty to fusion have demonstrated non-inferiority of ankle arthroplasty.[5,6] Furthermore, ankle arthrodesis has been shown to increase contact pressures in the subtalar, talonavicular, and calcaneocuboid articulations that commonly lead to degenerative changes in these adjacent joints, causing disability and the need for brace wear over time.[7,8] These findings have spurred the design overhaul and modernization of total ankle arthroplasty in recent years.

Total ankle arthroplasty design has undergone roughly 3 generations in the past 30 years.[9] The first generation was characterized by the use of cemented, highly constrained implants, which ultimately failed in the same way as their counterparts in the hip and knee did. The second generation included the widespread use of the Agility Total Ankle System prosthesis (DePuy, Warsaw, IN, USA). Distinct features of the Agility system included the need to establish a syndesmotic arthrodesis, as well as the use of an external fixator for distraction. The most recent, or third, generation has seen the arrival of worldwide use of the Scandinavian Total Ankle Replacement (STAR; Waldemar Link, Hamburg, Germany), INBONE Total Ankle System (Wright Medical Technology, Arlington, TN, USA), and Salto Talaris Anatomic Ankle Prosthesis (Tornier, Saint Ismier, France). Although numerous 3-component mobile bearing designs exist, the STAR is the only mobile bearing (3-component) design approved for use in the United States. Although, theoretically, a mobile bearing design allows for less stress and strain at the implant bone interface, no studies have demonstrated an increased rate of failure for a 2-component design versus a 3-component design.

This article describes the design features and technique tips for a newly released, fixed-bearing total ankle implant, the Cadence Total Ankle System (Integra LifeSciences, Plainsboro, NJ, USA).

CADENCE TOTAL ANKLE SYSTEM
Implant Design Features

- The tibial component is titanium alloy with 2 porous-coated pegs for bony ingrowth and a sharp posterior fin to seat the posterior aspect of the implant in the posterior portion of the resected tibia.
- The tibial component has an incisura on the lateral side to accommodate the natural position of the fibula without causing impingement on the implant.
- The polyethylene spacer is ultrahigh molecular-weight polyethylene, which is particularly resilient to wear over time.
- Posteriorly biased and anteriorly biased polyethylene inserts allow surgeons to correct anterior or posterior subluxation of the talus on the tibia.
- The talar component is cobalt chrome alloy with a porous-coated undersurface. The condylar design of the talar component conforms to the natural dome of the talus and does not have lateral or medial flanges. Therefore, there are no obstructions to viewing the implant bone interface on a lateral radiograph. This allows the surgeon to better evaluate for the presence of loosening or other implant interface issues (**Fig. 1**).
- Pin configurations placed during talar preparation are designed to minimize violation of the blood supply and thus the risk of avascular necrosis.
- Anterior and posteriorly biased polyethylene to help correct for sagittal plane malalignment or subluxation.

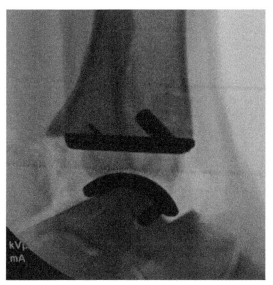

Fig. 1. Any loss of contact between the implant and subchondral bone (eg, secondary to aseptic loosening, fracture) is readily seen on subsequent films.

Clinical History

The determination of appropriate treatment of a patient with endstage tibiotalar arthritis should begin with a thorough history. Most patients will give some history of trauma to the affected ankle or other secondary cause of arthritis (eg, inflammatory or septic arthritis). Primary osteoarthritis is less common; in 1 study it accounted for only 10% of all cases of endstage tibiotalar arthritis.[10] Activity level and occupation should be noted to gauge and/or temper patient expectations regarding postsurgical outcome and function. Smoking and medical conditions, such as diabetes mellitus and peripheral vascular disease, factor into the discussion of risks and benefits with the patient.

Examination

The physical examination should begin with assessment of the patient's body habitus and gait. Evaluation of the skin over the affected extremity should be thorough. When determining existing range of motion, it is important to stabilize the hindfoot and midfoot because compensatory motion in these articulations may be present and give the impression of increased ankle range.[11] Any significant malalignment of the extremity above and below the ankle should be addressed either at the time of surgery or in a staged manner.

Radiographic Examination

Weightbearing radiographs are usually sufficient. Computed tomography and/or MRI can be used for evaluation of the extent of avascular necrosis, bone stock, and deformity.

Indications

Indications include debilitating, post-traumatic, degenerative, or inflammatory endstage tibiotalar arthritis.

Contraindications

Contraindications include active infection, large deformity, extensive talar avascular necrosis, loss of bone stock, severe neuropathy, or obesity.

Nonoperative Treatment

Nonoperative treatment may include activity modification, corticosteroid injections, shoewear customization/modification, or brace immobilization with an ankle foot orthoses (AFO) or Arizona brace.

Key Technique Pearls

- Surgery is performed under spinal anesthesia with an additional popliteal regional pain catheter for postoperative pain relief. The latter is placed by an anesthesiologist using ultrasound guidance and is removed postoperative day 3 by the patient at home.
- Make an anterior incision over ankle joint with enough length to allow for minimal tension edges and adequate contact of all guides or jigs. Retraction should be limited to cases in which it is necessary.
- Always identify and protect the superficial peroneal nerve after the skin incision. The extensor retinaculum can then be divided along its length.
- The interval between the tibialis anterior and the extensor hallucis longus is then exploited. The deep neurovascular bundle should be identified and retracted laterally. One can then cut down onto the bone underneath the tibialis anterior tendon and lift up flaps medially and laterally. With this technique, the neurovascular bundle and the extensor hallucis longus tendon are retracted laterally.
- In exposing the ankle joint, an anterior tibial cheilectomy can be performed to remove any offending osteophytes and allow one to properly visualize the joint surface. The extramedullary alignment guide is then mounted and secured with a noninvasive clamp proximally at the level of the tibial tubercle. The joint space evaluator can be placed in the ankle joint to give a rough guide of how far the alignment guide should come down for a proper tibial resection.
- Ensuring true anteroposterior (AP) and lateral views by getting perfect circles establishes the most accurate approximation of the different cuts. Any adjustments in height on the lateral view will result in a difference in the amount of medial malleolus taken. Therefore, it is advised to obtain an AP view of the ankle whenever a change in height on the lateral view is made (**Fig. 2**).
- Following the distal tibia cut, remove as much bone as possible in a controlled manner. It is possible to leave some bone for after the proximal talus cut is made; however, enough bone needs to be removed to not interfere with the talar cut guide seating correctly (**Fig. 3**).
- After both the distal tibia and proximal talar cuts are made, use the joint space evaluator to make sure that the minimum-sized implant will be able to be placed. If the evaluator cannot be placed into the rectangular space at this point, additional releases and/or bone resection need to be performed. A 2-mm additional resection cut guide is available to facilitate additional tibial resection.
- Both tibial and talar sizing are performed, and the respective bone surfaces are drilled and reamed as indicated.
- Avoid excessive dorsiflexion or axial load on the foot (ie, leaning forward on the foot) after the distal tibial cut is made. At this point, the malleoli are the only restraints to hyperdorsiflexion and will fracture with enough force.

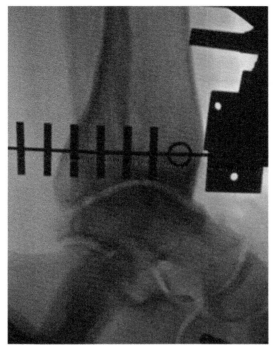

Fig. 2. Radiograph demonstrating a perfect circle and thus a true lateral view. The inferior end of the bars approximates the distal tibia cut surface.

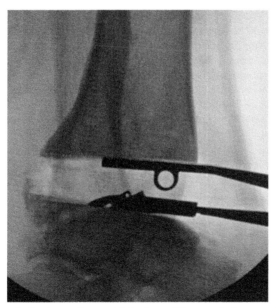

Fig. 3. As long as posterior bone does not interfere with correct placement of guides during talar preparation, it can be removed later in the procedure.

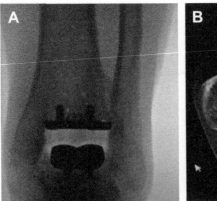
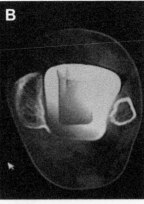
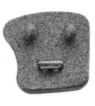

Fig. 4. On the AP view the implant appears to impinge on the fibula (*A*). This is a product of the design of the tibial implant, which is designed to anatomically contour to the axial surface of the distal tibia (*B, C*).

- While preparing the talus (proximal talus, posterior and anterior chamfers), taking one's eyes off the surgical field should be avoided. Although the Cadence technique was designed to minimize instrumentation changes, surgical error can still be introduced every time a new guide is mounted, pin exchanged, and so forth.
- When implanting the tibial component, ensure that the tray is being implanted parallel to the tibial cut surface.
- The tibial component will appear to be impinging on the fibula on an AP view. Unless the tibia is truly oversized, this is the product of the anatomic design of the tibial tray, which is wider anteriorly than posteriorly (**Fig. 4**).
- If anterior or posterior subluxation of the talar component on the tibial component is seen during trialing, consider the use of anteriorly or posteriorly biased polyethylene inserts. These will help centralize the talus on the tibia.
- The ankle should be splinted postoperatively to allow the incision to heal appropriately. Consider the use of a drain to prevent hematoma formation. There are no set guidelines about when weightbearing should be initiated.
- The authors' postoperative protocol involves 2 weeks in a nonweightbearing short-leg splint in neutral, followed by suture removal and weightbearing as tolerated in a fracture boot for an additional 4 wks. The boot may be removed for bathing and sleeping. Physical therapy and an over-the-counter ankle brace are initiated at 6-weeks postoperatively.

REFERENCES

1. Buckwalter JA, Saltzman C, Brown T. The impact of osteoarthritis: implications for research. Clin Orthop 2004;(427 Suppl):S6–15.
2. Salaffi F, Carotti M, Stancati A, et al. Health-related quality of life in older adults with symptomatic hip and knee osteoarthritis: a comparison with matched healthy controls. Aging Clin Exp Res 2005;17(4):255–63.
3. Arokoski MH, Haara M, Helminen HJ, et al. Physical function in men with and without hip osteoarthritis. Arch Phys Med Rehabil 2004;85(4):574–81.
4. Glazebrook M, Daniels T, Younger A, et al. Comparison of health-related quality of life between patients with end-stage ankle and hip arthrosis. J Bone Joint Surg Am 2008;90(3):499–505.

5. Saltzman CL, Mann RA, Ahrens JE, et al. Prospective controlled trial of STAR total ankle replacement versus ankle fusion: initial results. Foot Ankle Int 2009;30(7): 579–96.
6. Haddad SL, Coetzee JC, Estok R, et al. Intermediate and long-term outcomes of total ankle arthroplasty and ankle arthrodesis. A systematic review of the literature. J Bone Joint Surg Am 2007;89(9):1899–905.
7. Suckel A, Muller O, Herberts T, et al. Changes in Chopart joint load following tibiotalar arthrodesis: in vitro analysis of 8 cadaver specimens in a dynamic model. BMC Musculoskelet Disord 2007;8:80.
8. Jung H G, Parks BG, Nguyen A, et al. Effect of tibiotalar joint arthrodesis on adjacent tarsal joint pressure in a cadaver model. Foot Ankle Int 2007;28(1):103–8.
9. Cracchiolo A, Deorio JK. Design features of current total ankle replacements: implants and instrumentation. J Am Acad Orthop Surg 2008;16(9):530–40.
10. Valderrabano V, Horisberger M, Russell I, et al. Etiology of ankle osteoarthritis. Clin Orthop 2009;467(7):1800–6.
11. Dekker TJ, Hamid KS, Easley ME, et al. Ratio of range of motion of the ankle and surrounding joints after total ankle replacement: a radiographic cohort study. J Bone Joint Surg Am 2017;99(7):576–82.

Computed Navigation Guidance for Ankle Replacement in the Setting of Ankle Deformity

Feras J. Waly, MBBS, FRCS(C)[a,b,*], Nicholas E. Yeo, MBBS, FRCS[a,c,1],
Murray J. Penner, MD, FRCS(C)[d,1]

KEYWORDS

- Preoperative navigation • Patient-specific instrumentation • Total ankle arthroplasty
- Ankle deformity • PROPHECY • INBONE II • INFINITY

KEY POINTS

- Total ankle replacement represents a reliable treatment option for end-stage ankle arthritis.
- Patient-specific instrument guidance makes use of computed tomography scans to create an alignment guide that is specific to each patient's unique anatomy.
- Preoperative computed navigation guidance allows the surgeon to plan and execute the most appropriate bone cuts and implant positioning while correcting any associated deformities with reproducible results within 2° of the planned target alignment.
- Preoperative computed navigation guidance extends the indications for total ankle replacement.

INTRODUCTION

The use of preoperative imaging-derived patient-specific instrumentation[1] is not a new concept in total joint arthroplasty. It has been used in both total knee and hip arthroplasty

Disclosure Statement: No relationship with a commercial company that has a direct financial interest in subject matter or materials discussed in article or with a company making a competing product (F.J. Waly, N.E. Yeo). Consultants of Wright Medical Technology with no stock options (M.J. Penner).
[a] Department of Orthopaedic Surgery, St Paul's Hospital, 1081 Burrard Street, Vancouver, British Columbia V6Z 1Y6, Canada; [b] Department of Orthopedic Surgery, University of Tabuk, Tabuk 71491, Saudi Arabia; [c] Department of Orthopaedic Surgery, Singapore General Hospital, Outram Road, Singapore 169608, Singapore; [d] Department of Orthopedic Surgery, University of British Columbia, 3114 - 910 West 10th Avenue, Vancouver, British Columbia V5Z 1M9, Canada
[1] Present address: 1000-1200 Burrard Street, Vancouver, British Columbia V6Z 2C7, Canada.
* Corresponding author. 1000-1200 Burrard Street, Vancouver, British Columbia V6Z 2C7, Canada.
E-mail addresses: Feras.waly@mail.mcgill.ca; Feras.waly@gmail.com

Clin Podiatr Med Surg 35 (2018) 85–94
http://dx.doi.org/10.1016/j.cpm.2017.08.004
0891-8422/18/© 2017 Elsevier Inc. All rights reserved.

to improve accuracy of implant alignment and reduce operative times.[2–6] More recently, this technology has been implemented for use in total ankle replacement (TAR). Preoperative computed tomography (CT)-derived patient-specific guides (PROPHECY; Wright Medical Technology, Memphis, TN) have been developed for this purpose.[7–9]

Survivorship of TARs has yet to match that of knee and hip arthroplasty.[10] Despite advances and improving results, ankle deformities represent a great challenge to foot and ankle surgeons and are common in cases of end-stage ankle arthritis. Many surgeons have considered preoperative coronal plane deformity of greater than 10° a contraindication for a TAR due to the increased risk of instability, subluxation, and implant failure.[11,12] Doets and colleagues[13] reported increased failure rate in ankles with a preoperative coronal plane deformity greater than 10°, with an average survival rate of only 48% at 8 years. The unique anatomy and biomechanics of the ankle joint dictates that any minor malpositioning of the total ankle components results in an increase in peak pressures and decrease in contact areas. This contributes to polyethylene wear and subsequent implant failure.[14,15] In addition, compared with knee and hip arthritis, patients requiring TAR for end-stage ankle arthritis tend to be younger and relatively more active. As such, accuracy of component placement with restoration of mechanical and kinematic joint axes is of paramount importance for a good outcome following TAR.

Patient-specific instrument guidance makes use of CT or MRI scans of the ankle joint to create an alignment guide for each component of the implant that is specific to each patient's unique anatomy. This results in a custom fit of the implant, aligned with the appropriate axes as selected by the surgeon, which optimizes load distribution and avoids the need for sizing of implants intraoperatively. This, in turn, improves the accuracy and reproducibility of the implanted components and may potentially reduce the incidence of implant failure.[16,17]

SURGICAL TECHNIQUE

The PROPHECY preoperative navigation alignment guide is the first described system used in the foot and ankle to provide preoperative implant position planning. This guide is intended for use with the INFINITY Total Ankle System (Wright Medical Technology) and the INBONE II Total Ankle System (Wright Medical Technology).

These systems are indicated for use in patients with end-stage ankle arthritis who are suitable for a TAR. Contraindications for use include active infection, vascular insufficiency, inadequate bone stock, neuropathic joints, severe neuromuscular conditions, and excessively high-demand patients.

Preoperative Planning

Preoperatively, after reviewing the weightbearing radiographs of the foot and ankle (Fig. 1), the patient undergoes a CT scan following the PROPHECY Ankle CT Scan protocol. This ideally includes hip-to-foot CT scout images, although knee-to-foot images are acceptable.[18] High-resolution scans of the knee, foot, and ankle are required.

These scans are then used to produce a 3-dimensional (3D) computer bone model with anatomic reference points on the tibia and talus. In addition, the CT scan is used to assess preoperative coronal plane, sagittal plane, and rotational deformity, and identify the mechanical and anatomic axes on both coronal and sagittal images. This allows the surgeon to choose the tibial mechanical or anatomic axis for positioning of the tibial component, taking into account any deformity that may be present in the tibia. The 3-D model also allows the medial and lateral gutter angles of the tibial plafond to be identified, and these are used to determine axial rotation.

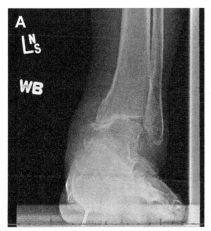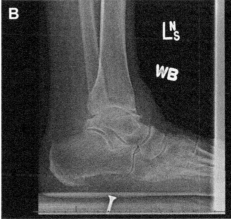

Fig. 1. Preoperative weightbearing AP (*A*) and lateral (*B*) radiographs of the left ankle.

Using computer software, the implant is then overlaid onto the 3-D model, then positioned and sized as follows. The tibial component is set perpendicular to the long axis selected by the surgeon (mechanical or anatomic). Axial rotation of the tibial component is typically set by the bisection of the medial and lateral gutter angles, although this can be altered by surgeon choice. The coronal plane position of the tibial implant is set to match the medial corner of the tibial plafond and the sagittal plane position set to the anterior edge of the tibia. The talar component is set to align to the bottom of the foot when in neutral standing position. This determination may be augmented by referencing a standing lateral radiograph of the ankle. Size of the talus implant is selected to maximize bone coverage while minimizing implant overhang. Axial rotation of the talar component is set by the bisection of the medial and lateral talar side walls, although final positioning is determined intraoperatively. The resection level of the talus is set such that the implant dome matches the natural talar dome. Once the desired preoperative alignment is set on the computer model, the PROPH-ECY guides are then produced based on the preoperative plan (**Fig. 2**). These guides will position the guide pins that hold the cutting jigs, ensuring the tibial and talar resections are aligned to the preoperative plan.

Surgical Approach

The patient is placed supine on the operating table with a thigh tourniquet and a bump under the ipsilateral buttock to maintain the leg in neutral rotation. A standard longitudinal anterior incision is made, following the extensor hallucis longus (EHL) tendon, starting approximately 7 cm above the ankle joint and carried to the talonavicular joint to give a wide exposure. The extensor retinaculum is incised along the lateral edge of the EHL tendon. Care should be taken to preserve the medial dorsal cutaneous nerve, which may cross over the distal incision lateral to medial, and to identify the neurovascular bundle proximal to the ankle joint, just medial and deep to the EHL tendon. The neurovascular bundle is retracted laterally together with the EHL and extensor digitorum longus tendons, and the tibialis anterior (TA) tendon is retracted medially. All dissection is carried lateral to the TA tendon sheath and care taken not to violate it, ensuring it remains enclosed in the sheath throughout. The ankle joint capsule is then incised and detached from the tibia and talus using sharp dissection to expose the ankle joint.

On entering the ankle joint, all existing anterior tibia and dorsal talar osteophytes must be preserved. Loose bodies noted on the preoperative scans should be

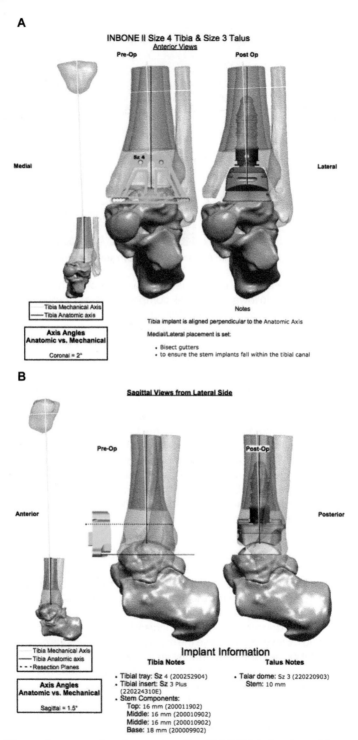

Fig. 2. A CT scan demonstrating the preoperative PROPHECY planning with assessment of the mechanical and anatomic axis, components alignment, and resection level on coronal (*A*) and sagittal (*B*) views.

removed. Any remaining periarticular soft tissue overlying the distal tibia and dorsal talar neck should be meticulously excised. A periosteal elevator in combination with electrocautery may be used for this. This is a crucial step that allows the PROPHECY alignment guides to sit flush on the bone. Any remnant soft tissue may tilt the implant and prevent anatomic seating of the patient-specific guide.

Tibial Preparation

The tibial guide is oriented onto the distal tibia until a "surface match" fit is found. It should be noted that the guides are designed to fit in only one proper location. If the guides do not sit flush on the tibia, make sure to clean off any remaining soft tissue covering the bone before driving any pins into the tibia. Once the guide is properly seated, it is pinned in position. A pin is placed through the vertical hole in the center handle of the guide to serve as a coronal alignment cue. An anteroposterior (AP) fluoroscopic image is then taken to confirm the tibia guide is in the correct orientation. Once the desired fit and alignment are confirmed, a total of 4 pins are placed through the guide into the tibia. The PROPHECY guide is removed and the coronal sizing guide is then inserted through the pins. Fluoroscopic AP and lateral views are then obtained to verify the tibial resections. On the AP view, the coronal profile of the tibial component as well as the tibial resection line can be assessed. On the lateral view, the flexion/extension angle of the planned tibial resections can be verified.

The tibial corner drill is then used to bicortically drill both proximal corners of the tibia. The coronal sizing guide is then replaced with the tibial resection guide of the appropriate size, as determined by the preoperative plan. An oscillating saw is then used to make the tibial resections through the proximal, medial, and lateral slots of the resection guide. Completion of the posterior cortical resection is done with a reciprocating saw for greater control. The anterior part of the resected tibia bone is then removed. This allows enough exposure for the talar preparation.

Talar Preparation

The foot is placed in plantarflexion for maximum exposure of the talar dome. Again, the area of the talar neck and dome where the talar guide rests should be free of all soft tissue, including any residual cartilage that may still be present. The PROPHECY talar guide is then oriented to the talar surface in the "surface match" position. If the talar guide does not sit properly, check that there is no remaining soft tissue on the talar surface and increase the plantar flexion of the foot to optimize exposure of the talar surface. Similarly, once the proper position is obtained, the guide is fixed to the talus with pins. The proximal/distal location and flexion/extension angle of the talar component can now be verified under fluoroscopy. On the lateral view, the proximal talar resection is approximately 2 mm proximal to the top of the horizontal pin.

The PROPHECY alignment guide is then removed and replaced with the talar resection guide. An oscillating saw is then used to complete the talar resection. The resected talar dome is then removed. A corner chisel is then used to finish off the residual bone cuts in the proximal corners of the resected tibia. The remaining resected tibia bone cut is then removed with the aid of a bone removal screw.

Trialing and Implantation of Components

The tibial tray trial is placed through the remaining 2 tibial pins into the resected joint space. Optimal AP tibial coverage and implant positioning can be assessed fluoroscopically. There is an option of a standard or long AP-sized tibial component. Once tibial trial position is confirmed, broaching of the tibial peg is performed.

The talar dome trial is then inserted and the polyethylene insert trial is engaged into the tibial component trial. Fluoroscopic lateral images at this juncture are critical to confirm that the posterior edge of the talar trial matches that of the residual talus, thereby establishing congruence of the talar dome. Fluoroscopic AP images are used to minimize any medial or lateral overhang of the talar component to avoid gutter impingement. The ankle is moved through repeated range of motion to ensure the talar component achieves axial alignment with the tibial component. Once the trialing of component is satisfactory, pins are placed in the talar trial component, and these are used to position the talar chamfer guide, allowing the talar chamfer resections to be completed. Trialing is again carried out, this time with the final talar trial, and care is taken to ensure appropriate coronal plane position. Once confirmed, the talar peg holes are drilled. The final tibial and talar components are then implanted.

Trialing of different polyethylene (PE)-bearing thicknesses is then carried out. In cases with no or minimal deformity, good ligamentous balance is typically present and the bearing thickness is selected based on a good balance of stability and range of motion. In cases with significant preoperative deformity, the bearing trial is a crucial step. We have found that preoperative navigation guidance allows the surgeon to perform individual bony cuts and insertion of the tibial and talar components before any soft tissue balancing procedures. This workflow is very useful, as it allows the surgeon to optimize the balancing procedures to be used, because the actual biomechanics of the ankle can be taken into account.

If the ankle tilts into varus with insertion of the trial PE bearing, a deltoid ligament release or a distal-sliding medial malleolar osteotomy may be necessary, and may be readily added. Care must be observed, however, because this will increase the joint space, and a thicker PE bearing may be needed. Because the range of PE-bearing thicknesses is limited, it is prudent for the surgeon to consider this possibility preoperatively and ensure that the tibial resection level is not excessive. If the joint space may become too wide with medial releases, or if the lateral malleolus is blocking the talus from tilting back to neutral alignment, then a fibular shortening osteotomy or fibular tip resection with gutter widening may be needed (**Fig. 3**). Lateral ligament

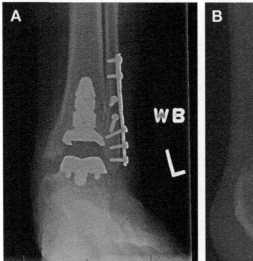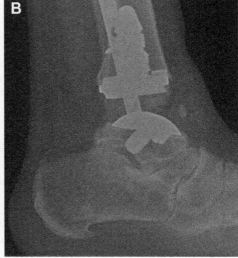

Fig. 3. Postoperative weightbearing AP (*A*) and lateral (*B*) radiographs of the left ankle.

reconstruction with a modified Brostrom procedure is commonly used in varus deformity cases. In severe varus, the posteromedial structures are often tight, including the posterior tibial (PT) tendon. Transfer of the PT tendon to peroneus brevis should be considered in such severe cases.

In cases with valgus deformity, joint laxity is more prevalent and even greater care is needed in preoperative planning to ensure that excessive tibial bone is not resected. If this occurs, it may be possible, particularly when using the INFINITY system, to have insufficiently thick PE-bearing options, because 12-mm thickness is the maximum. Severe valgus cases with overt deltoid ligament insufficiency present a major challenge. Deltoid ligament reconstruction techniques have been published, and may be attempted, but long-term results are lacking, and outcomes may be unpredictable. In less severe cases, lateral malleolar distal-sliding osteotomies or lateral ligament releases may help achieve balance. However, in valgus cases, foot realignment to a neutral plantigrade position is the most important concept, and may require multiple flatfoot reconstruction procedures.

CLINICAL RESULTS WITH PROPHECY PREOPERATIVE NAVIGATION SYSTEM

TAR has experienced innovation and improving outcomes over the past decades. Still, orthopedic surgeons are faced with a predicament when dealing with preoperative ankle deformities. One must note that component alignment and soft tissue balancing are major concerns during a primary TAR when dealing with deformity.[19–21] It is crucial to obtain a good component placement that is reproducible, while correcting the coronal plane deformity in TAR to decrease the incidence of increased peak pressures, eccentric wear, component loosening, and premature failure of TAR.[22,23] However, recent reports show encouraging outcomes following TAR in patients with preoperative deformity with an emphasis on deformity correction and proper components alignment.[21,24]

The theoretic benefits of preoperative navigation using patient-specific guides are improved accuracy and reproducibility of component alignment and facilitation of a greater understanding of the patient's deformity, thereby improving deformity correction. This in turn may decrease the need for corrective osteotomies, reduce the learning curve through more efficient presurgical planning, decrease operative time, and thereby potentially lower cost.[25–27]

The literature is still lacking substantial evidence; however, early preliminary reports on the use of preoperative computer-assisted guidance for TAR are encouraging. Adams and colleagues[28] reported on the accuracy of component placement to improve outcome and implant survival. They showed the coronal and sagittal angulation of the tibial saw cut made with conventional Scandinavian Total Ankle Replacement (STAR) instruments to be similar, in a matched cadaveric setting, to cuts guided by a computerized navigation system.

Preoperative computer-assisted guidance for TAR has made the surgical technique more reproducible. Berlet and colleagues[7] investigated the accuracy and reproducibility of CT-guided patient-specific guides in a cadaveric model. Average variation between planned and actual postoperative implant placement was less than 2° and 1.4 mm in all specimens tested. Component placement was analyzed using multiple cameras to determine the position of infrared marker arrays on the distal tibia and talus, followed by software processing. The investigators concluded that surgical plans and guides provided reliable and reproducible placement of TAR implants, which was similar to the modern total knee replacement navigation systems. Similarly Hsu and colleagues[8] reported on the use of PROPHECY preoperative navigation guides, which aided in obtaining neutral alignment in 100% of their 42 patients.

The accuracy and reproducibility of implant position with patient-specific guides for TAR were investigated in 44 patients by Daigre and colleagues[9] In a multicenter retrospective study, they showed that in 79.5% of patients, the postoperative implant position of the tibia corresponded to the preoperative plan of the tibia within 3° of the intended target, within 4° in 88.6% of patients, and within 5° in 100% of patients. The tibial component coronal size was correctly predicted in 98% of cases, whereas the talar component was correctly predicted in 80% of cases.

However, clinical outcomes data are limited to a single case report. Hanselman and colleagues[29] reported acceptable radiographic and clinical outcome at 8 months in a 54-year-old man with preoperative varus ankle deformity of 29°.

The senior author has used PROPHECY preoperative patient-specific guides for all primary INBONE II cases since 2012 and all INFINITY cases since 2014, apart from those in which accurate CT scans could not be obtained due to technical factors, such as excessive metallic hardware. Coronal plane deformity greater than 10° in either varus or valgus was present in 30% of cases, with a maximum deformity of 34° varus. The use of patient-specific guides has proven extremely valuable in improving preoperative planning, determination of the need for, and selection of, additional realignment and soft tissue balancing procedures, and reduced operative time for complex cases. Formal publication of the results of these cases is pending, although to date there have been no revision surgeries and there are no pending revisions. Patients are followed clinically with biennial radiographs and none have demonstrated any deformity recurrence (talar tilt >2°). Overall, the addition of patient-specific preoperative guidance has dramatically improved the ease and reliability of deformity correction in these complex cases.

SUMMARY

TAR now represents a reliable treatment option for end-stage ankle arthritis. Attention has gradually shifted from the appropriateness of TAR and the specific type of TAR system, and is now focused on proper positioning of the implants. Recent advances in technology have led to better understanding the 3-D ankle anatomy and associated deformities. The use of preoperative computer-assisted guidance now allows reliable placement of the TAR components in anatomic position, potentially expanding the indications for TAR to include ankle deformities that were previously considered a relative contraindication. Preoperative computer-assisted guidance allows the surgeon to plan and execute the most appropriate bone cuts and implant positioning while correcting any associated deformities with reproducible results within 2° of the planned target alignment. Further clinical studies are needed to examine clinical outcomes of preoperative navigation in patients with preoperative ankle deformity.

REFERENCES

1. Aad G, Abbott B, Abdallah J, et al. Combined measurement of the Higgs Boson Mass in pp Collisions at sqrt[s]=7 and 8 TeV with the ATLAS and CMS experiments. Phys Rev Lett 2015;114(19):191803.
2. Ast MP, Nam D, Haas SB. Patient-specific instrumentation for total knee arthroplasty: a review. Orthop Clin North Am 2012;43(5):e17–22.
3. Boonen B, Schotanus MG, Kort NP. Preliminary experience with the patient-specific templating total knee arthroplasty. Acta Orthop 2012;83(4):387–93.
4. Hsu AR, Gross CE, Bhatia S, et al. Template-directed instrumentation in total knee arthroplasty: cost savings analysis. Orthopedics 2012;35(11):e1596–600.

5. Thienpont E, Schwab PE, Fennema P. Efficacy of patient-specific instruments in total knee arthroplasty: a systematic review and meta-analysis. J Bone Joint Surg Am 2017;99(6):521–30.

6. Haglin JM, Eltorai AE, Gil JA, et al. Patient-specific orthopaedic implants. Orthop Surg 2016;8(4):417–24.

7. Berlet GC, Penner MJ, Lancianese S, et al. Total ankle arthroplasty accuracy and reproducibility using preoperative CT scan-derived, patient-specific guides. Foot Ankle Int 2014;35(7):665–76.

8. Hsu AR, Davis WH, Cohen BE, et al. Radiographic outcomes of preoperative CT scan-derived patient-specific total ankle arthroplasty. Foot Ankle Int 2015;36(10): 1163–9.

9. Daigre J, Berlet G, Van Dyke B, et al. Accuracy and reproducibility using patient-specific instrumentation in total ankle arthroplasty. Foot Ankle Int 2017;38(4): 412–8.

10. Bartel AF, Roukis TS. Total ankle replacement survival rates based on Kaplan-Meier survival analysis of National Joint Registry Data. Clin Podiatr Med Surg 2015;32(4):483–94.

11. Haskell A, Mann RA. Ankle arthroplasty with preoperative coronal plane deformity: short-term results. Clin Orthop Relat Res 2004;(424):98–103.

12. Wood PL, Prem H, Sutton C. Total ankle replacement: medium-term results in 200 Scandinavian total ankle replacements. J Bone Joint Surg Br 2008;90(5):605–9.

13. Doets HC, Brand R, Nelissen RG. Total ankle arthroplasty in inflammatory joint disease with use of two mobile-bearing designs. J Bone Joint Surg Am 2006; 88(6):1272–84.

14. Fukuda T, Haddad SL, Ren Y, et al. Impact of talar component rotation on contact pressure after total ankle arthroplasty: a cadaveric study. Foot Ankle Int 2010; 31(5):404–11.

15. Kakkar R, Siddique MS. Stresses in the ankle joint and total ankle replacement design. Foot Ankle Surg 2011;17(2):58–63.

16. Schwarzkopf R, Brodsky M, Garcia GA, et al. Surgical and functional outcomes in patients undergoing total knee replacement with patient-specific implants compared with "off-the-shelf" implants. Orthop J Sports Med 2015;3(7). 2325967115590379.

17. Harrysson OL, Hosni YA, Nayfeh JF. Custom-designed orthopedic implants evaluated using finite element analysis of patient-specific computed tomography data: femoral-component case study. BMC Musculoskelet Disord 2007;8:91.

18. Technology WM. PROPHECY® pre-operative navigation guides ankle CT scan protocol. 2014. Available at: http://www.wmtemedia.com/ProductFiles/Files/PDFs/008380_EN_LR_LE.pdf. Accessed May 3, 2017.

19. Choi WJ, Kim BS, Lee JW. Preoperative planning and surgical technique: how do I balance my ankle? Foot Ankle Int 2012;33(3):244–9.

20. Queen RM, Adams SB Jr, Viens NA, et al. Differences in outcomes following total ankle replacement in patients with neutral alignment compared with tibiotalar joint malalignment. J Bone Joint Surg Am 2013;95(21):1927–34.

21. Hobson SA, Karantana A, Dhar S. Total ankle replacement in patients with significant pre-operative deformity of the hindfoot. J Bone Joint Surg Br 2009;91(4): 481–6.

22. Hsu AR, Haddad SL, Myerson MS. Evaluation and management of the painful total ankle arthroplasty. J Am Acad Orthop Surg 2015;23(5):272–82.

23. Jonck JH, Myerson MS. Revision total ankle replacement. Foot Ankle Clin 2012; 17(4):687–706.

24. Kim BS, Choi WJ, Kim YS, et al. Total ankle replacement in moderate to severe varus deformity of the ankle. J Bone Joint Surg Br 2009;91(9):1183–90.
25. Reb CW, Berlet GC. Experience with navigation in total ankle arthroplasty. Is it worth the cost? Foot Ankle Clin 2017;22(2):455–63.
26. Angthong C, Adams SB, Easley ME, et al. Radiation exposure in total ankle replacement. Foot Ankle Int 2014;35(11):1131–6.
27. Simonson DC, Roukis TS. Incidence of complications during the surgeon learning curve period for primary total ankle replacement: a systematic review. Clin Podiatr Med Surg 2015;32(4):473–82.
28. Adams SB Jr, Spritzer CE, Hofstaetter SG, et al. Computer-assisted tibia preparation for total ankle arthroplasty: a cadaveric study. Int J Med Robot 2007;3(4):336–40.
29. Hanselman AE, Powell BD, Santrock RD. Total ankle arthroplasty with severe preoperative varus deformity. Orthopedics 2015;38(4):e343–6.

The Use of Decellularized Human Placenta in Full-Thickness Wound Repair and Periarticular Soft Tissue Reconstruction

An Update on Regenerative Healing

Stephen A. Brigido, DPM[a],*, Scott C. Carrington, DPM[a],
Nicole M. Protzman, MS[b]

KEYWORDS

- Amniotic membrane • Extracellular matrix • Growth factors • Placenta
- Regenerative healing

KEY POINTS

- The intrinsic properties of connective tissue matrix enhance the healing process by providing a scaffold for cell attachment, allowing the release of endogenous growth factors and cytokines.
- Micronized placenta has numerous applications in the foot and ankle, including the treatment of deep tunneling wounds and augmentation of various soft tissue and bone procedures.
- Although basic science and clinical studies show promising results, additional research is needed to better understand the applications and therapeutic benefits of amniotic tissue in regenerative medicine.

Disclosure statement: Dr S.A. Brigido serves on the surgery advisory board for Alliqua. He also serves as a consultant for Stryker. Alliqua and Stryker had no knowledge or influence in study design, protocol, or data collection. Drs S.C. Carrington and N.M. Protzman have nothing to disclose.

[a] Foot and Ankle Reconstruction, Foot and Ankle Department, Coordinated Health, 2775 Schoenersville Road, Bethlehem, PA 18017, USA; [b] Clinical Integration Department, Coordinated Health, 3435 Winchester Road, Allentown, PA 18104, USA
* Corresponding author.
E-mail address: drsbrigido@mac.com

INTRODUCTION

Injuries of the foot and ankle are a common source of pain and disability. They are especially challenging when the healing process is prolonged or incomplete. Consequently, investigators have begun searching for alternative treatment strategies. With advances in tissue engineering, decellularized placenta has been suggested as a means to achieve more rapid and complete healing.

SCIENCE AND APPLICATION
Structure

Decellularization is the process whereby cells are removed from soft tissue scaffolds to eliminate antigens that can cause an increased inflammatory process or a rejection response. It has been well described that controlling inflammation is the cornerstone to minimizing fibrosis and scar tissue formation. In order for the body to enter a pathway of *regenerative* healing that is defined as healing with minimal to no scar, 3 key events must occur. First, cells must proliferate within the soft tissue scaffold. Second, vascularization of the soft tissue scaffold must occur. Finally, the scaffold must transition into the host tissue in a functional form. Decellularized, allogenic soft tissue scaffolds may, when processed and handled correctly, provide an ideal platform for regenerative healing to occur. In 2003, Hopper and colleagues[1] first described the use of a decellularized human placenta as a vascular scaffold for large tissue engineered implants. The human placenta is a complex organ that facilitates a symbiotic relationship between mother and fetus. The placenta is rich in growth factors and, equally as important, contains a rich amount of extracellular matrix (ECM) components.[2] Since then, an increased understanding of tissue healing and regeneration has allowed scaffolds like decellularized placenta to be used in areas such as wound healing and soft tissue reconstruction.

Function

The way in which cells interact with the ECM often dictates the healing response within injured tissue. Decellularized human placental connective tissue matrix (CTM) (Interfyl, Alliqua BioMedical, Yardley, PA) contains key extracellular proteins important for cell adhesion, such as fibronectin and laminin. Pashuck and colleagues[3] demonstrated that human dermal fibroblasts, human epidermal keratinocytes, and human dermal microvascular endothelial cells adhere and proliferate on CTM. When these cells proliferate and adhere to the CTM, the stimulated cells release growth factors, such as vascular endothelial growth factor and fibroblast growth factor.[3] These same bench top data demonstrated that placental CTM support the migration of endothelial cells, prompt endothelial cell attachment, and, finally, promote the formation of endothelial tube formation.[3] Pashuck and colleagues[3] further hypothesized that CTM may act as a scaffold that can replace abnormal ECM in damaged tissue that allows endogenous cells to accelerate healing and regeneration.[3] Healing and regeneration occur through suppression of the M1 macrophage and increased expression of the M2 macrophage. The M2 macrophage is responsible for tissue remodeling. Improved and accelerated tissue remodeling coupled with endothelial tube formation and cellular migration provides an opportunity for placental CTM to be a pathway for regenerative healing.

Wound Care

Complex, nonhealing wounds present a significant challenge for foot and ankle surgeons. The environment of nonhealing wounds is wrought with deficits in the ECM, elevated concentrations of proinflammatory cytokines and metalloproteinases, and decreased growth factor activity.[4,5] Consequently, many complex wounds fail to respond to standard treatment modalities. Chronic inflammation within the wound supports uncontrolled proinflammatory macrophages. The combination of an abnormal ECM and excess M1 macrophages does not support an environment for healing and ultimately needs to be interrupted for closure to occur.

The aforementioned bench top data presented by Pashuck and colleagues[3] demonstrate that placental CTM may be a scaffold that can help stop the uncontrolled cycle of inflammation and abnormal ECM. By providing a stable environment for cell attachment, endothelial cell formation, and ultimately the release of endogenous growth factors, CTM establishes a healthy cascade for regeneration and ultimately epithelialization.[3]

The surgical technique for the application of CTM to full-thickness wounds is very similar to the application of other allograft products. The key to successful application is aggressive debridement of the wound to eliminate all bioburden. Once all nonviable fibrinous tissue is removed, the scaffold is placed on the wound in an evenly distributed fashion. Alternative, the surgeon can use the flowable scaffold through a syringe or a particulate form out of a vial.

Plantar Fasciitis

The underlying pathologic processes of plantar fasciitis are poorly understood, though most histologic studies report degenerative changes at the plantar fascia enthesis. The most common pathologic features are deterioration of collagen fibers, increased secretion of ground substance proteins, focal areas of fibroblast proliferation, and increased vascularity.[6,7] Thus, plantar fasciitis seems to be more of a degenerative process than an isolated inflammatory process.

Plantar fasciitis is widely considered a self-limited condition[8] with spontaneous resolution of symptoms occurring in approximately 80% of patients within 12 months.[9] Initial conservative management includes a variety of therapies, including activity modification, icing, nonsteroidal antiinflammatory drugs, orthotics, splinting, and physical therapy. Approximately 10% of patients will fail to improve with conservative care, and chronic heel pain greatly impacts quality of life for many patients before resolution.[10] For patients who fail conservative treatment, other modalities have been described in the literature, including extracorporeal shock wave therapy, platelet-rich plasma injections, corticosteroid injections, and surgical interventions.

A localized corticosteroid injection has generally been considered an effective, relatively long-term solution and, therefore, a mainstay of nonsurgical treatment.[11,12] Despite their widespread use, the risks associated with corticosteroid injections include fat pad atrophy and plantar fascia rupture.[13] The degenerative pathophysiology of plantar fasciitis also calls into question the use of corticosteroids for long-term relief.

In contrast, human amniotic tissues are well known for their healing characteristics. Studies have shown that the biomechanical properties of amniotic membranes promote soft tissue healing by enhancing regenerative stages while limiting scarring and inflammation.[14,15] In a study by Zelen and colleagues,[16] patients with refractory plantar fascial pain showed a statically significant improvement in American Orthopedic Foot and Ankle Society scores over an 8-week period with micronized dehydrated amniotic/chorionic membrane allograft heel injections. More recently, Hanselman and colleagues[17] demonstrated that the use of cryopreserved human amniotic membrane was as safe and efficacious as corticosteroids when injected into patients with plantar heel pain. **Fig. 1** shows a plantar fascia injection with decellularized human placental CTM (Interfyl, Alliqua Biomedical).

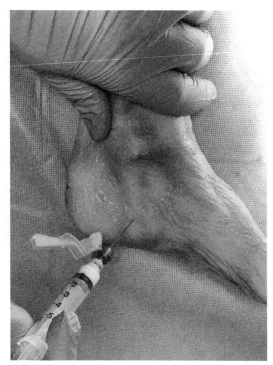

Fig. 1. Plantar fascia injection with Interfyl.

Tendons

Tendon healing occurs in a series of stages.[18] Initially a fibroblastic splint is formed. During this time, the tendon is in its weakest state. During the second stage, there is an increase in paratenon vascularity and collagen proliferation. During stage 3, approximately 3 full weeks from the start of the healing process, the collagen fibers align longitudinally. During this time, the tendon shows a moderate increase in strength and controlled passive range of motion can be initiated. The fourth and final phase begins at 4 weeks, whereby the tendon has increased strength and can tolerate active mobilization.[18]

Use of amniotic membrane for tendon repair has the potential to decrease inflammation and tissue adhesion early in the tendon healing process. In animal models, investigators have confirmed the ability of amniotic cells to increase the number of proliferating tendon reparative cells,[18] improve tendon strength,[16,19] decrease adhesion formation,[19,20] and differentiate into tendonlike material.[19,21] Despite these encouraging results, there is a paucity of clinical evidence.

In a sheep model, amniotic epithelial cells were applied to calcaneal tendon defects and demonstrated the presence of amniotic cells up to 1 month after implantation.[20] Furthermore, the study showed that amniotic cells have the ability to increase the number of proliferating tendon reparative cells, which are important for collagen products and, in turn, tendon healing.[20] Similar results were found by Kueckelhaus and colleagues[19] who transected and primarily repaired the Achilles tendon in 2 groups of rats. One group received a saline injection, whereas the other received an injection of amnion-derived cellular cytokine solution (ACCS) in carboxy-methyl cellulose

(CMC) gel. The treatment group that received the ACCS in CMC had improved breaking strength, tensile strength, and yield strength early in the reparative process.[19] This finding is important, as increased healing earlier on in the process will allow for earlier rehabilitation of the involved tendon and may lead to improved functional outcomes.

In 2009, Ozböulük and colleagues[21] presented the results in rabbit models comparing 3 treatment groups. Each group underwent division of the flexor fibularis tendon with repair using a modified Kessler technique. One group underwent tendon repair (control group), one group underwent tendon repair with amniotic membrane application (treatment group 1), and the final group underwent tendon repair with application of periosteal autograft (treatment group 2).[21] Biomechanically, the group treated with tendon repair and application of periosteal autograft showed the greatest strength. Adhesion formation in both the amniotic membrane group and the periosteal autograft group were found to yield greater outcomes than the control group.[21] Although this study was conducted using a rabbit model,[21] it suggests that the application of an amniotic membrane in a tendon repair model can decrease adhesion formation and, presumably, postoperative pain.

Demirkan and colleagues[22] reported similar findings with respect to adhesion formation in a chicken model. They reported on the use of amniotic membrane in hand surgery. Three groups were compared: tendon repair alone, tendon repair with tendon sheath repair, and tendon repair with application of an amniotic membrane. The adhesions in group 3 (application of an amniotic membrane) were significantly reduced. The investigators also noted that 3 months following repair, in group 3, there was no evidence of the amniotic membrane remained, indicating full incorporation and conversion of the cells into tendinous structure.[22] These findings are further supported by Barboni and colleagues[23] who extracted amniotic epithelial cells and coincubated those cells with explanted tendons or primary tenocytes of fetal or adult calcaneal tendon. In the coincubated group of amniotic cells with fetal-derived tendon or tenocytes, the investigators reported high differentiation of the amniotic cells into tendon-like material, exhibiting a highly organized structure.[23]

Figs. 2 and **3** illustrate the injection of CTM (Interfyl, Alliqua BioMedical) for tendon sheath repair and tendon repair, respectively. **Fig. 4** shows closure of the tendon sheath.

Bone

Autogenous bone graft is the gold standard for the reconstruction of bone defects and is the preferred adjunctive tissue for arthrodesis procedures. Be that as it may, there is a limited supply of autogenous bone as well as a risk of donor site morbidity. As a result, bone graft substitutes have been developed. Examples include silicone, polymethyl methacrylate, hydroxyapatite, demineralized bone matrix, and tricalcium phosphate.[24–26] These materials help to augment boney procedures, while avoiding graft procurement.

Until recently, bone autograft was the only material available with osteogenic, osteo-inductive, and osteo-conductive properties. Advancement in bioengineering has introduced a means of biologically augmenting skeletal fractures and arthrodesis procedures.

Daniels and colleagues[27] studied the efficacy and outcomes of purified recombinant human platelet-derived growth factor BB homodimer combined with beta-tricalcium phosphate (rhPDGF-BB/β-TCP-collagen) in ankle and hindfoot arthrodesis. They showed complete fusion at 24 weeks in 84% of patients treated with rhPDGF-BB/β-TCP-collagen versus 65% of patients treated with autograft. Additionally, successful

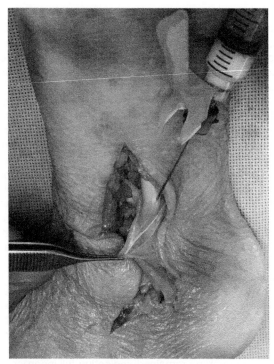

Fig. 2. Tendon sheath injection with Interfyl.

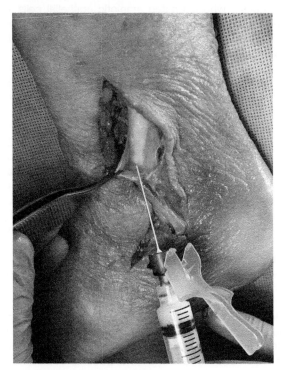

Fig. 3. Injection of Interfyl onto a tendon repair.

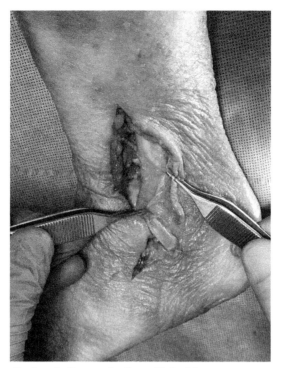

Fig. 4. Tendon sheath closed after application of Interfyl.

clinical outcomes at 52 weeks were achieved in 91% of rhPDGF-BB/β-TCP-collagen–treated patients versus 78% of autograft patients.[27] Platelet-derived growth factor (PDGF) has been shown to stimulate blood vessels and play a key role in promoting tissue repair.[28] The angiogenic properties of PDGF, combined with strong mitogenic chemotactic effects on mesenchymal cells, play a central role in the early phases of the healing cascade.[28]

Starecki and colleagues[29] studied the healing potential of amniotic tissue augmentation in a rat model. They created a critical-sized femoral gap in 3 separate groups: no treatment specimens, specimens treated with commercially available bone graft, and, finally, specimens treated with bone graft and amniotic tissue. The study demonstrated statistically significant potential for amniotic membrane products to provide bridging of bone defects.[29]

In 2012, Zhong and colleagues[30] showed that placenta-derived mesenchymal stem cells (PDMSCs) have a promising advantage for bone tissue engineering. In their study, PDMSCs offered advantages in availability, biological activities, cell adhesion, immunogenicity, cytokine production, and osteoblastic differentiation.[30]

The surgical technique for applying placental CTM is very straightforward for the surgeon. Each joint to be fused is prepared by denuding the articular surface and subchondral plate using curettage, and the subchondral bone is fenestrated using a 0.062-mm Kirschner wire. Approximately 2.5 cm^3 of cancellous autogenous bone is harvested from either the ipsilateral calcaneal body or proximal tibia and mixed with 100 mg of allogeneic, decellularized, particulate human placental CTM. The combined 2.5 mL/100 mg mixture is placed in each joint to be fused. Appropriate hardware is placed around the fusion as the surgeons deems necessary.

SUMMARY/DISCUSSION

During healing, the body may deposit excess fibrous collagen at the site of injury. Current measures for treating excess scarring and adhesions on traumatized tendons and chronic wounds include bovine collagen wraps, sheets of hyaluronic acid, hydroscopic polymer-based barriers (eg, polyethylene glycol), xenograft sheets, and numerous other agents to assist in healing. In published clinical studies, none of these approaches have been shown to consistently reduce the incidence of adhesions or scar formation following repair of the injured extremity. As described earlier, decellularized human placental CTM has been shown to support regenerative healing in the clinical setting[16,17,27] and through bench top data.[3] Regenerative healing includes cellular proliferation across the scaffold, endothelial penetration, and ultimately a transition to functional host tissue. This transition to functional tissue allows for an environment that has minimal scar tissue that closely resembles that of the preinjured state.

REFERENCES

1. Hopper RA, Woodhouse K, Semple JL. Acelluarization of human placenta with preservation of the basement membrane: a potential matrix for tissue engineering. Ann Plast Surg 2003;51:598–602. Available at. https://insights.ovid.com/pubmed?pmid=14646657.
2. Choi JS, Kim BS, Kim JD, et al. In vitro cartilage tissue engineering using adipose-derived extracellular matrix scaffolds seeded with adipose-derived stem cells. Tissue Eng A 2012;18:80–92. Available at. https://www.ncbi.nlm.nih.gov/pmc/articles/PMC3246412/.
3. Pashuck ET, Mao Y, Kim K, et al. A human placenta-derived decellularized connective tissue matrix (CTM) supports cellular functions involved in wound healing processes. Symposium on Advanced Wound Care. 2016.
4. Falanga V, Grinnel F, Gilchrest B, et al. Experimental approaches to chronic wounds. Wound Repair Regen 1995;3:132–40. Available at. http://onlinelibrary.wiley.com/doi/10.1046/j.1524-475X.1995.30205.x/abstract;jsessionid=8DDACCD771C11D82889D3C90F2C8DBD7.f02t03.
5. Foy Y, Li J, Kirsner R, et al. Analysis of fibroblast defects in extracellular matrix production in chronic wounds. J Am Acad Dermatol 2004;50:P168. Available at. http://www.jaad.org/article/S0190-9622(03)04002-7/pdf.
6. Lemont H, Ammirati K, Usen N. Plantar fasciitis: a degenerative process (fasciosis) without inflammation. J Am Podiatr Assoc 2003;93:234–7. Available at. http://www.drkristaarcher.com/wp-content/uploads/2012/09/plantarfasciitis.pdf.
7. Jarde O, Diebold P, Havet E, et al. Degenerative lesion of the plantar fascia: surgical treatment by fasciectomy and excision of the heel spur. A report on 38 cases. Acta Orthop Belg 2003;69:274–6. Available at. https://s3.amazonaws.com/academia.edu.documents/41953815/09-jarde-vernois-.pdf?AWSAccessKeyId=AKIAIWOWYYGZ2Y53UL3A&Expires=1502818495&Signature=JTh%2F9zzjxBPgAFPs9fIjKtL5NaQ%3D&response-content-disposition=inline%3B%20filename%3DDegenerative_lesions_of_the_plantar_fasc.pdf.
8. Buchbinder R. Clinical practice. Plantar fasciitis. New Engl J Med 2004;350:2159–66. Available at. http://www.nejm.org/doi/full/10.1056/NEJMcp032745.
9. Wolgin M, Cook C, Graham C, et al. Conservative treatment of plantar heel pain: long-term follow up. Foot Ankle Int 1994;15:97–102. Available at. http://journals.sagepub.com/doi/abs/10.1177/107110079401500303?url_ver=Z39.88-2003&rfr_id=ori:rid:crossref.org&rfr_dat=cr_pub%3dpubmed.

10. Irving DB, Cook JL, Young MA, et al. Impact of chronic plantar heel pain on health-related quality of life. J Am Podiatr Med Assoc 2008;98:283–9. Available at. http://www.japmaonline.org/doi/abs/10.7547/0980283?code=pmas-site.

11. Genc H, Saracoglu M, Nacir B, et al. Long-term ultrasonographic follow-up of plantar fasciitis patients treated with steroid injection. Joint Bone Spine 2005;72:61–5. Available at. http://www.sciencedirect.com/science/article/pii/S1297319X04000752.

12. Porter MD, Shadbolt B. Intralesional corticosteroid injection versus extracorporeal shock wave therapy for plantar fasciopathy. Clin J Sport Med 2005;15:119–24. Available at. https://insights.ovid.com/pubmed?pmid=15867552.

13. Acevedo JI, Beskin JL. Complications of plantar fascia rupture associated with corticosteroid injection. Foot Ankle Int 1998;19:91–7. Available at. http://journals.sagepub.com/doi/abs/10.1177/107110079801900207?url_ver=Z39.88-2003&rfr_id=ori:rid:crossref.org&rfr_dat=cr_pub%3dpubmed.

14. Niknejad H, Peirovi H, Jorjani M, et al. Properties of the amniotic membrane for potential use in tissue engineering. Eur Cell Mater 2008;15:88–99. Available at. http://www.ecmjournal.org/papers/vol015/vol015a07.php.

15. Adzick NS, Lorenz HP. Cell, matrix, growth factors, and the surgeon. The biology of scarless fetal wound repair. Ann Surg 1994;220:10–8. Available at. https://www.ncbi.nlm.nih.gov/pmc/articles/PMC1234281/.

16. Zelen CM, Poka A, Andrews J. Prospective, randomized, blinded, comparative study of injectable micronized dehydrated amniotic/chorionic membrane allograft for plantar fasciitis–a feasibility study. Foot Ankle Int 2013;34:1332–9. Available at. http://journals.sagepub.com/doi/abs/10.1177/1071100713502179?url_ver=Z39.88-2003&rfr_id=ori:rid:crossref.org&rfr_dat=cr_pub%3dpubmed.

17. Hanselman AE, Tidwell JE, Santrock RD. Cryopreserved human amniotic membrane injection for plantar fasciitis: a randomized, controlled, double-blind pilot study. Foot Ankle Int 2014;36:151–8. Available at. http://journals.sagepub.com/doi/abs/10.1177/1071100714552824?url_ver=Z39.88-2003&rfr_id=ori:rid:crossref.org&rfr_dat=cr_pub%3dpubmed.

18. Fitzgerald RH. Management of acute and chronic tendon injury. In: McGlamry's comprehensive textbook of foot and ankle surgery. 4th edition. Philadelphia: Lippincott Williams & Wilkins; 2014. p. 1549–80.

19. Kueckelhaus M, Philip J, Kamel RA, et al. Sustained release of amnion-derived cellular cytokine solution facilitates achilles tendon healing in rats. EPlasty 2014; 14:e29. Available at. https://www.ncbi.nlm.nih.gov/pmc/articles/PMC4124919/.

20. Muttini A, Mattioli M, Petrizzi L, et al. Experimental study on allografts of amniotic epithelial cells in calcaneal tendon lesions of sheep. Vet Res Commun 2010;34:117–20. Available at. https://link.springer.com/article/10.1007%2Fs11259-010-9396-z.

21. Ozböülük S, Ozkan Y, Oztürk A, et al. The effects of human amniotic membrane and periosteal autograft on tendon healing: experimental study in rabbits. J Hand Surg Eur Vol 2010;35:262–8. Available at. http://journals.sagepub.com/doi/abs/10.1177/1753193409337961?url_ver=Z39.88-2003&rfr_id=ori:rid:crossref.org&rfr_dat=cr_pub%3dpubmed.

22. Demirkan F, Colakoglu N, Herek O, et al. The use of amniotic membrane in flexor tendon repair: an experimental model. Arch Orthop Trauma Surg 2002;122:396–9. Available at. https://link.springer.com/article/10.1007%2Fs00402-002-0418-3.

23. Barboni B, Russo V, Curini V, et al. Achilles tendon regeneration can be improved by amniotic epithelial cell allotransplantation. Cell Transpl 2012;21:2377–95. Available at. http://journals.sagepub.com/doi/abs/10.3727/096368912X638892?url_ver=Z39.88-2003&rfr_id=ori:rid:crossref.org&rfr_dat=cr_pub%3dpubmed.

24. Nauth A, McKee MD, Einhorn TA, et al. Managing bone defects. J Orthop Trauma 2011;25:462–6. Available at. https://insights.ovid.com/pubmed?pmid=21738065.

25. Murugan R, Ramakrishna S. Development of nanocomposites for bone grafting. Comp Sci Technol 2005;65:2385–406. Available at. http://opac.vimaru.edu.vn/edata/E-Journal/2005/Composite%20science%20and%20technology/Vol65is15-16/bai%2011.pdf.

26. Bucholz RW, Carlton A, Holmes RE. Hydroxyapatite and tricalcium phosphate bone graft substitutes. Orthop Clin North Am 1987;18:323–34. Available at. http://europepmc.org/abstract/med/3561978.

27. Daniels TR, Younger AS, Penner MJ, et al. Prospective randomized controlled trial of hindfoot and ankle fusions treated with rhPDGF-BB in combination with β-TCP-collagen matrix. Foot Ankle Int 2015;36:739–48. Available at. http://bcfootandankle.com/wp-content/uploads/2016/03/Injectible-PDGF.full_.pdf.

28. Alvarez RH, Kantarjian HM, Cortes JE. Biology of platelet-derived growth factors and its involvement in disease. Mayo Clin Proc 2006;81:1241–57. Available at. http://www.mayoclinicproceedings.org/article/S0025-6196(11)61237-8/fulltext.

29. Starecki M, Schwartz JA, Grande DA. Evaluation of amniotic-derived membrane biomaterial as an adjunct for repair of critical sized bone defects. Adv Orthop Surg 2014;2014:572586. Available at. http://downloads.hindawi.com/journals/aos/2014/572586.pdf.

30. Zhong ZN, Zhu SF, Yuan AD, et al. Potential of placenta-derived mesenchymal stem cells as seed cells for bone tissue engineering: preliminary study of osteo-blastic differentiation and immunogenicity. Orthopedics 2012;35:779–88. Available at. https://www.healio.com/orthopedics/journals/ortho/2012-9-35-9/%7Bdbf57f5b-0b05-4296-b10f-fb5bd664f72a%7D/potential-of-placenta-derived-mesenchymal-stem-cells-as-seed-cells-for-bone-tissue-engineering-preliminary-study-of-osteo blastic-differentiation-and-immunogenicity.

Treating Charcot Arthropathy Is a Challenge

Explaining Why My Treatment Algorithm Has Changed

Lawrence DiDomenico, DPM[a],*, Zachary Flynn, DPM, AACFAS[a],
Michael Reed, DPM[h]

KEYWORDS

- Charcot • Neuroarthropathy • Charcot reconstruction • Staged approach to Charcot
- Surgical algorithm for Charcot • Charcot challenges • Diabetic reconstruction
- Diabetic limb salvage

KEY POINTS

- The background, pathophysiology, and the conservative care options available for the Charcot patient are discussed.
- Foot and ankle surgeons attempting reconstruction and ultimate salvage of Charcot deformed limbs face challenges.
- The staged protocol used by the senior author, experiences, and outcomes of this approach are discussed, as well as the benefits versus a single-staged approach.

INTRODUCTION

First described in 1703 by Sir William Musgrave[1] but brought into recognition by Jean-Martin Charcot in 1868,[2] osteo-neuroarthropathy was most commonly caused by tabes dorsalis (**Figs. 1–13**). Because of this, Charcot himself dubbed the term tabetic foot in 1883 even after obtaining his eponym.[1] However, tabetic foot has been replaced by the term diabetic foot as the leading cause of Charcot neuroarthropathy. With a reported prevalence of 0.1% to 0.4%[1,3] in the general population, Charcot neuroarthropathy prevails in up to 3.0% in patients with diabetes.[4]

[a] St. Elizabeth Medical Center, 8175 Market Street, Youngstown, OH 44512, USA; [b] Northside Medical Center, 500 Gypsy Lane, Youngstown, OH 44512, USA
* Corresponding author.
E-mail address: ld5353@aol.com

Clin Podiatr Med Surg 35 (2018) 105–121
http://dx.doi.org/10.1016/j.cpm.2017.08.012
0891-8422/18/© 2017 Elsevier Inc. All rights reserved.

podiatric.theclinics.com

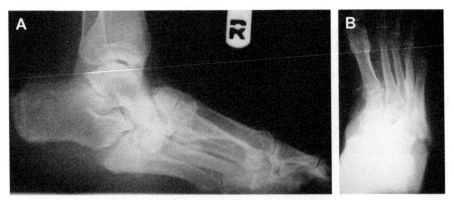

Fig. 1. Case 1: (*A*, *B*) Preoperative anteroposterior (AP) and lateral radiographs. The lateral radiograph demonstrates the sequela of an equinus contracture resulting in a negative calcaneal inclination angle and a dislocation of the midfoot. The AP view demonstrates a midfoot overload secondary to a metatarsal adducts, resulting in overload of the lateral column, resulting in a long-standing diabetic foot ulcer that lead to osteomyelitis.

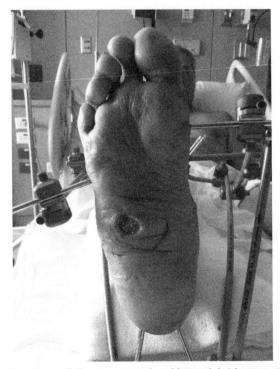

Fig. 2. Case 1: A clinical view following wound and bone debridement. An osteotome was used to fracture, or perform, an osteotomy of the midfoot and harvest bone for a culture and pathologic testing. Note the skin wrinkles in the midfoot as the foot was manipulated and anatomically reduced, resulting in offloading the wound or ulcer. Negative pressure therapy was used for granulation of the wound while the patient received 6 weeks of intravenous antibiotics.

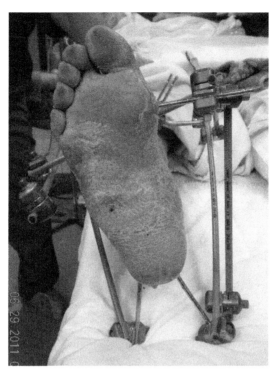

Fig. 3. Case 1: Postoperative well-healed wound following a posterior muscle lengthening, bone debridement, reduction of the deformity into anatomic alignment, application of external fixation, negative pressure therapy, and intravenous antibiotics. The wound has healed well and the soft tissue envelope is optimized for reconstructive surgery.

PATHOPHYSIOLOGY

Charcot neuroarthropathy is characterized by the gradual progressive destruction of bone and joints,[2] yet the exact pathophysiology is still unknown. The disorder involves episodes of active and inactive phases[5] with a rapid onset of swelling, increased temperature, and sometimes discomfort. Typically, many patients with Charcot neuroarthropathy have long-standing diabetes for more than 10 years and often have good perfusion.[1] Classic hypotheses, along with several recent theories, are discussed.[1–3,6]

The neurovascular theory, or French theory, was proposed by Charcot in 1868.[5,7] In his study of more than 5000 subjects, he suggested that autonomic neuropathy was the main cause because of changes in spinal trophic centers of the anterior horn.[7] This autonomic neurogenic loss of vasomotor tone, or autosympathectomy, results in arteriovenous shunts opening into Volkmann and haversian canals.[1] An approximately 30% to 60% increased blood flow into bone allows a hyperemic demineralization of bone to occur with osteoclastogenesis. With minerals being washed out and uncontrolled stimulation of osteoclasts, bone becomes osteopenic with a high propensity for breakdown in the insensate foot.[1,2] Evidence of a vascular-inflammatory connection is seen with Charcot neuroarthropathy secondary to revascularization.[8]

A competitive philosophy is the neurotraumatic, or German theory, relating to unperceived trauma.[1] Reportedly, diabetic patients have a higher incidence of fractures compared with persons without diabetes.[9–11] Sensory neuropathy permits repetitive microtrauma resulting in inconspicuous stress fractures and joint destruction.

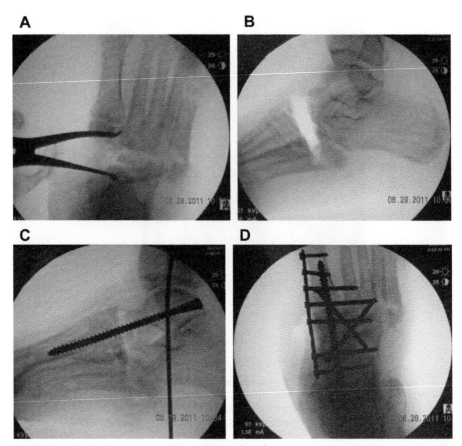

Fig. 4. Case 1: (*A*, *B*) Intraoperative radiographs of an internal amputation resecting the diseased Charcot bone and osteomyelitis, providing a surgical, as well as a medical, cure via intravenous antibiotics. (*C*, *D*) Intraoperative radiographs of deformity reduction with rigid internal fixation. C demonstrates a full-threaded solid 6.5 bolt realigning Meary's angle. D demonstrates the midfoot aligned into anatomic alignment with a 6.5 solid full-threaded bolt coupled by independent screw fixation and plating. Note that talar first metatarsal angle is re-established. The bone voids were packed with bone graft, giving the midfoot an excellent chance to successfully fuse. By performing the bony resection, placing the foot into anatomic alignment, and obtaining an arthrodesis, the deforming force is removed and the patient should experience a permanent long-term correction.

Persistent degeneration becomes permanently deformed, showing the importance of neural control of skeletal homeostasis.[12] Obesity has been speculated to overload joints and accelerate the formation of Charcot. Although it is associated with Charcot, elevated body-mass indices do not increase the risk of acute Charcot neuroarthropathy.[3] Additionally, some case reports followed diabetic neuropathic patients who underwent successful bariatric surgery who developed acute Charcot.[13] It was concluded that, even though diabetes had gone into remission, the end-organ damage it had caused (eg, peripheral neuropathy) did not change. These patients became more ambulatory, increasing the stress to their numb feet.

Excessive osteoclastic activity has been reported during acute Charcot neuroarthropathy.[7] Osteoclastogenesis is mediated by receptor activator of nuclear factor

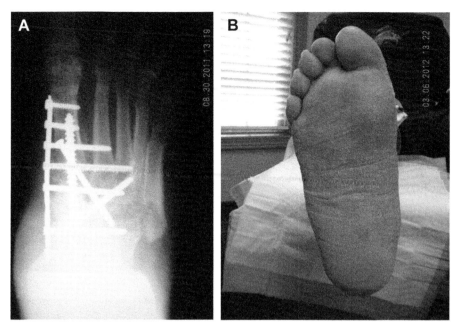

Fig. 5. Case 1: (*A*) A 6-year postoperative AP view demonstrating good anatomic alignment and a successful arthrodesis. (*B*) A 6-year postoperative clinical view demonstrating good anatomic alignment, a well-healed wound, and the deforming force permanently removed, leading to a good long-term outcome.

kappa-β ligand (RANKL) and modulated by the RANKL–osteoprotegerin balance. If this equilibrium is disrupted, osteoclastic activity will have no negative feedback and osteopenia will arise.[1] However, a study[14] showed a RANKL-independent pathway revealing osteoclastic precursor cells primed with aggressive behavior in patients with Charcot neuroarthropathy. This pathway was filled with proinflammatory factors that stimulated osteoclast formation, separate from RANKL.[1,15] Prolonged inflammation and osteolysis induced by Charcot neuroarthropathy resembles that of rheumatoid arthritis and periodontal disease.[2] Advanced glycation end products from hyperglycemia also affect cortical bone by increasing RANKL activation and osteoblast apoptosis.[16]

Leptin has been found to be related to bone mass.[9] However, in the diabetic patient, leptin hormone levels are increased, which in turn substantially reduces bone mass. This is a result of a receptor mutation, blocking the hormone and its signaling. Solid organ transplantation has likewise been reported with Charcot neuroarthropathy.[17–21] One study showed 5% of simultaneous pancreatic-renal transplant patients acquired Charcot neuroarthropathy within their first post-transplant year.[17] Situations such as this may be due in part by heavy corticosteroid use, impaired renal function, or nutritional deficiency that cause bone resorption.[22]

A combination theory has moreover been described by blending the different processes. For example, the autonomic neuropathy causes bone demineralization because the sensory neuropathy is amenable to uncompensated microtrauma.[1] During the acute stages of the disease, Charcot neuroarthropathy typically is made up of soft bone, whereas later stages show hard, brittle bone. In a recent study comparing trabecular quality histologically, Charcot patients demonstrated thin trabeculae with

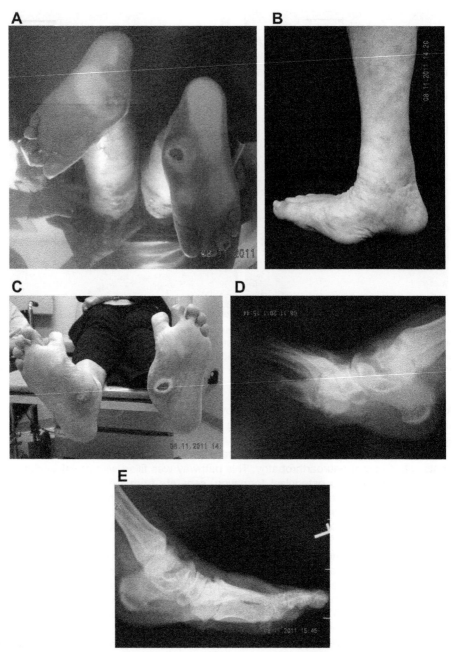

Fig. 6. Case 2: (*A*) Bilateral midfoot Charcot arthropathy. Unfortunately the patient has experienced chronic bilateral diabetic foot ulcers secondary to the midfoot deformity, re-sulting in a chronic ulceration with osteomyelitis, making the patient susceptible to limb loss bilaterally. Note the abnormal weightbearing pattern of the feet, leading to chronic ul-ceration and infection. (*B, C*) Significant deformities of bilateral feet causing long-standing deformities and chronic ulcers with osteomyelitis. (*D, E*) Radiographs demonstrating a lack of integrity throughout midfoot with significant Charcot arthropathy of both feet.

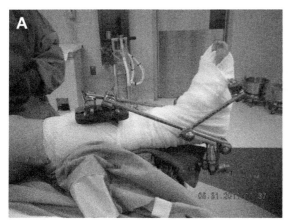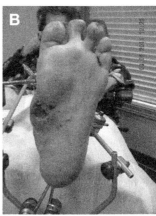

Fig. 7. Case 2: (*A*) Intraoperative view of the patient having a compressive bandage applied, following the posterior muscle lengthening, bone debridement for cultures and pathologic testing, manipulation and reduction of the foot deformity, application of an external fixator, wound negative pressure therapy, and a compressive postoperative bandage. (*B*) A postoperative visit demonstrating a wound that is granulating nicely with no evidence of infection. Note the foot is anatomic alignment and stable allowing the wound to be offloaded with easy access to the wound.

inflammatory infiltrates and hypervascular myxoid tissue.[2] Other publications indicate that bone in diabetic patients is weaker with 1 study comparing young diabetic animal models with older nondiabetic animals. The results found similar structural changes in both groups and suggested that diabetes may increase the normal aging process.[23] Interestingly, osteoporotic bone, whether in a geriatric or a long-standing diabetic patient, will generally be stiff but brittle with increased risk for fracturing, whereas poorly mineralized bone in a pediatric patient will be very flexible, which decreases the risk of fracture.

CONSERVATIVE CARE

Whether surgical or nonoperative, the treatment objective for Charcot neuroarthropathy is to achieve a plantigrade foot with bony stability.[2] Traditionally, nonoperative treatment has been used with offloading devices, including total contact casting, Charcot restraint orthotic walkers (CROWs), and bracing.[1,6,24,25] Although some patients will have a debilitating fixed deformity or gross instability that may not respond to bracing or casting alone,[5] 1 investigator noted that 60% of patients with midfoot Charcot neuroarthropathy attained a desirable outcome without surgical intervention.[26] Serial radiographs are important to carefully observe further fragmentation in the acute stage or coalescence with adequate immobilization.

Because a rigid bony deformity is very likely in patients with Charcot collapse, evidence clearly shows that effective offloading reduces the likelihood of ulceration, as well as amplifies the odds of healing an ulcer.[27] Pressure relief is essential. In a small study,[28] ulceration rates of subjects with and without Charcot neuroarthropathy were followed using custom orthotic treatment. Before orthotics, the ulceration rate of Charcot subjects was 73% (compared with 31% of non-Charcot). After 1-year follow-up, rates reduced dramatically to 9.8%, which was statistically significant. Yet in the acute phase, a total contact cast is preferred. Duration of offloading is guided by clinical assessment of edema, erythema, and skin temperature changes.[1]

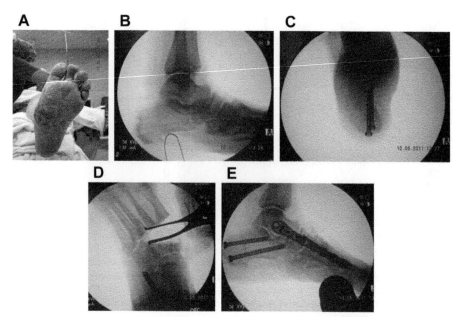

Fig. 8. Case 2: (*A*) Clinical view of the foot right after the external fixator is removed. Note the wound completely healed and soft tissue envelope is intact with no stress or inflammatory effects of the disease process, resulting in the patient being optimized for surgical reconstruction. (*B*) Lateral intraoperative view demonstrating a percutaneous calcaneal osteotomy with a Gigli saw. (*C*) Intraoperative view of a calcaneal axial view demonstrating medialization of the calcaneus with 2 large cancellous screws for fixation. (*D*) Intraoperative view demonstrating an internal amputation, an aggressive bone resection of the diseased midfoot removing the pathologic bone. (*E*) Intraoperative lateral view following a gastrocnemius recession, a percutaneous calcaneal displacement osteotomy, an aggressive bone resection (an internal amputation) with realignment and rigid internal fixation. Note the increase in the calcaneal inclination angle, the well-aligned Meary's angle and a recreation of the arch off-loading ulceration and the original deformity.

Conservative treatment involving pressure-offloading devices can be effective biomechanically. On the pharmacologic aspect, bisphosphonate mechanism of action is used to decrease osteoclastic resorption and increase osteoblastic activity. A small study[29,30] was conducted comparing alendronate against placebo. Both treatment groups were managed with standard offloading regimens. Although there was no report on clinical differences, investigators noticed a statistically significant decline in markers of bony turnover. As an alternative to bisphosphonates, calcitonin can be used in patients with renal insufficiency.[1] Vitamin D levels should also be tested because this deficiency can aid in bone loss.[22]

However, unless acute Charcot neuroarthropathy is well-managed from beginning, most patients will have some instability or bony prominence that will be amenable to surgical intervention. In cases that are mismanaged or missed, reconstruction or amputation may need to be pursued. The argument of limb salvage versus primary amputation has yet to be settled, and evidence-based outcomes on the matter are sparse. To truly evaluate reconstruction versus amputation, one must consider that 85% of patients with a diabetic foot ulceration and/or deformity report being unable to ambulate independently, which limits their physical activity and quality of life.[31] The claim that primary amputation leads to shorter recovery and quicker return to

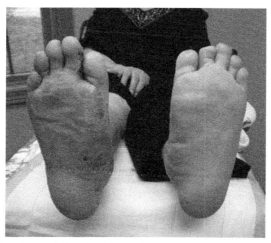

Fig. 9. Case 2: A clinical view following bilateral, reconstructive, staged surgery of both feet. The patient's left foot was done initially, followed by the right foot. The feet are in more normal anatomic alignment, therefore eliminating the underlying pathologic condition, creating plantigrade, stable feet, resulting in long-term correction of a severe deformities that are free of ulceration and infection.

function with a prosthesis is grim. Only 47% to 67% of patients who undergo a primary amputation secondary to ischemia or ulceration are able to rehabilitate to independent function with their prosthesis.[32] Additionally, patients with a primary lower extremity amputation secondary to diabetes have been shown to have a 30% increase

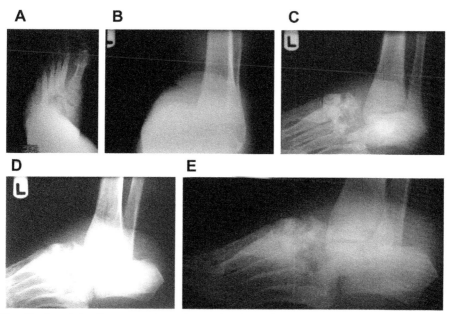

Fig. 10. Case 3: (*A–E*) Preoperative radiographs of significant Charcot arthropathy involving the tibial talar joint, talar calcaneal joint, and the midfoot.

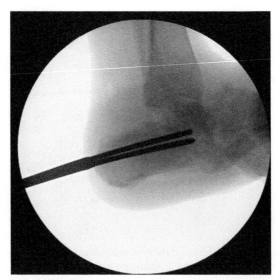

Fig. 11. Case 3: An intraoperative lateral view of half pins placed in the calcaneus from posterior to anterior preceded by half pins placed in the tibia and midfoot. Placing the half pins in the calcaneus from posterior to anterior provides advantages because this allows more contact of half pin to bone and provides more leverage when attempting the get the ankle out of equinus. Two pins provide the surgeon more control of the hind foot in all 3 cardinal planes.

incidence of depression.[33] Mortality rates following primary amputation reach up to 40% 1-year postoperatively, and 80% after 5 years.[34]

From an economic standpoint, collected data showed the mean reimbursement for all Medicare services for a patient with diabetic foot ulceration was $16,700 in 2008, compared with $36,500 for someone who underwent a major lower extremity amputation.[35] Recent retrospective cost analysis has shown that lifelong costs for major lower extremity amputations can average $509,275, which is about 3 times higher than the costs for patients who undergo reconstruction.[32] Given the high level of morbidity and excessive costs associated with amputation, reconstruction by a multidiscipline team has been shown to be effective.[31–33,35,36]

SURGICAL RECONSTRUCTION

Surgical reconstruction and salvage is typically offered when conservative care has failed. Additional indications are ulceration or preulcerative lesions, osteomyelitis, and pain. In recent studies, the anatomic locations of surgical reconstructions have been changing. The most common locations requiring surgical intervention based on a 54-year review (1960–2014) for patients with Charcot was the midfoot (43.5%), followed by the ankle (33.8%). During the past 5 years, the most common locations requiring surgical intervention were the hindfoot (41.6%), followed by the ankle (38.4%). Although midfoot and hindfoot Charcot have a higher rate of occurrence than the ankle, the midfoot is more amenable to bracing and other nonoperative treatment methods than cases in which the ankle is affected. Additionally, surgeons are quicker to address the posterior muscle group, reducing plantar pressures and halting midfoot breakdown.[37]

Various fixation techniques have been described and analyzed, including internal fixation, external fixation, combination techniques, and superconstructs. One study discussed a comparison between internal and external fixation techniques for surgical

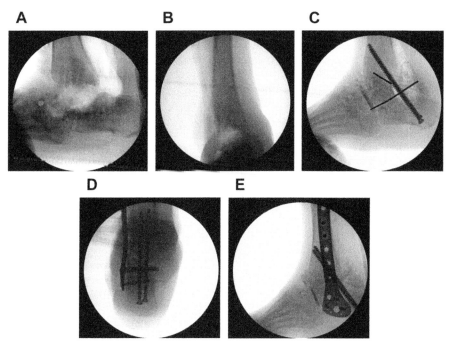

Fig. 12. Case 3: (*A*, *B*) Intraoperative view following an internal amputation of the diseased and osteomyelitis bone. (*C–E*) Intraoperative views following the takedown of the fibula. The distal cortical cancellous block of the distal fibula was used as an inlay graft and the remaining fibula was put into a bone mill and, coupled with allogenic bone, was packed tightly into the bone voids. Fixation is provided through 2 fully threaded solid large cancellous screws and a femoral locking plate.

reconstruction of the foot and ankle in patients who are not infected. The addition of the circular external fixation device did not affect the overall limb salvation rate or complication rate. Overall, the data continue to be too inconclusive to recommend any form of fixation over another.[36,38] (See discussion of fixation options, in this issue.)

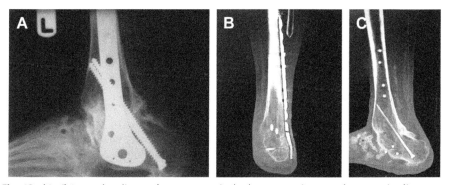

Fig. 13. (*A–C*) Lateral radiograph postoperatively demonstrating good anatomic alignment and a solid bony union to the tibial talar, talar calcaneal, and midfoot. The computed tomography scan demonstrates a bony union of the hind foot and ankle with anatomic alignment. The bone graft successfully replaced the osteomyelitis and Charcot bone, allowing for good bony union.

The decision on whether to approach surgical reconstruction in a single-stage or a multistage approach is usually based on patient deformity and surgeon preference. Studies have been inconclusive about whether reconstruction during the acute phase is beneficial. Typically, patients requiring reconstruction have had ulcerations, osteomyelitis, or significant deformity. It was these characteristics that led the senior author to use a staged approach.

TRANSITION TO STAGED PROTOCOL

The complexity of the Charcot patient is often underestimated. This patient population includes some the most ill patients a foot and ankle surgeon will encounter. Quite often these patients have uncontrolled diabetes, peripheral vascular disease, obesity, hypertension, cardiac issues, and smoke tobacco.[4,6,8,11,25] Complete lifestyle modification and medical optimization is required to sustain a biologic environment for healing and recovery. Referrals to multiple medical specialties are necessary to correct the metabolic imbalances. Endocrinology, vascular surgery, and infectious disease are involved in virtually all Charcot reconstructions.

In addition to the systemic disease processes, these patients have significant deformity of the foot and ankle, often with severe ulcerations. Data have shown that postoperative complications and infection rates decrease if surgery can be postponed until wounds are closed.[3] Additionally, a recent study by Sohn and colleagues[39] found that those patients with Charcot deformity and an ulceration were 12 times more likely to undergo a major amputation then those without ulceration. The value of a healthy soft tissue envelope was another driving force to the staged protocol. Controlling the edema, resolving wounds, and proper moisturizing techniques can help reduce future wound complications and decrease the patients' risk for limb loss. In a study by Aragón-Sánchez and colleagues,[40] major amputation was recommended for 2 cases of severe Charcot deformity complicated by osteomyelitis. Four major steps were used for limb salvage:

1. Partial removal of infected bone by curettage
2. Culture-guided postdebridement antibiotic treatment
3. Bed rest before placement in a total contact cast
4. Stabilization of the unstable foot using a total contact cast with an opening for performing wound care and to check healing.

Although this protocol was successful, most patients requiring reconstruction have significant deformity and soft tissue breakdown. Treatment with an external fixator is more amenable to providing stability and addressing wounds and soft tissues complications, while also forcing patient compliance.

Staged Reconstruction

First stage of the reconstruction surgery

After medical optimization and appropriate consultations, the patient undergoes the first stage of reconstruction. Typically, this patient population experiences an equinus contracture of the posterior muscle group. A Silfverskiöld test is performed once the patient is under anesthesia to determine if the equinus contracture is gastrocnemius or gastrocnemius and soleus in nature. Based on the results of the Silfverskiöld test, a gastrocnemius recession is performed either open or endoscopically.[35] Once the posterior muscle group is lengthened, the surgeon can mobilize the deformity much more easily, reduce the deformity, and maintain the ankle out of equinus. The posterior muscle lengthening procedure is mandatory to obtain an adequate reduction. Attention is directed to the wound and the deformity. This generally consists of wound debridement or excision, and bone debridement if bone is exposed. Bone is sent for pathologic testing, as well as for cultures and Gram stain. Next, manipulation and reduction of the deformity is performed and stabilization of the deformity in anatomic alignment is accomplished with the use of a multilevel external fixator. Application of negative pressure therapy is applied to the wound to assist with wound treatment. All affected bone or bone that has been exposed, is debrided, biopsied, and sent for cultures. Depending on the deformity, an osteotome, rongeur, or curette is used to harvest and resect bone. If the deformity is flexible, then the deformity is reduced and placed into anatomic alignment and fixated with an external fixator. If the deformity is rigid, an osteotome is used to weaken and/or fracture through the deformity, bone is harvested for pathologic testing and cultures, and then manipulation and reduction of the deformity into a more normal alignment is performed. A multilevel external fixator (typically, we use a bar-clamp external fixator) is used to maintain correction in the desired anatomic position. The external fixator provides stability and maintains the deformity in anatomic alignment; therefore, offloading the wound by correcting the deformity that was causing the wound. Additionally, it provides easy access to the wound. The patients are admitted to the hospital and an infectious disease consultation, as well as social service consultation are made in attempt for skilled nursing. Bone and tissue cultures are evaluated and followed by an infectious disease specialist who typically manages any infection with intravenous antibiotic therapy. During the postoperative course, the inflammatory markers are evaluated. The inflammatory markers often mirror the wound. Because of the reduction of the deformity, as well as the offloading of the wound, along with negative pressure therapy, the wound typically goes on to heal uneventfully, closing the soft tissue envelope. In cases of large and more complicated wounds, negative pressure therapy is performed weekly and advanced wound care and/or split-thickness skin grafting is used in attempt to close the wound. Edema control with bandaging is performed at every dressing change to prevent soft tissue complications, as well as pin tract infection. Appropriate moisturizing is also implemented to improve soft tissue integrity. Once wound healing is achieved, preparation for next definitive stage of the surgical reconstruction begins. It has been the senior author's experience that it is best to maintain anatomic alignment of the foot and ankle and to allow several weeks for the soft tissue envelope to remodel and mature so that the soft tissues are optimized for the definitive stage of the reconstructive surgery. Additionally the inflammatory markers are followed by an infectious disease specialist to assess and to identify when the patient is most optimized for the definitive and reconstructive surgery (**Figs. 1–3**).

Second definitive stage of the surgical reconstruction
This stage consists of removing the external fixator and thoroughly cleansing the entire lower extremity using peroxide, as well as providing a sterile preparation of the limb, before the surgical reconstruction. Once a good sterile preparation and draping is accomplished, all incisions are made full thickness in an attempt to preserve the soft tissue envelope. Aggressive bone resection eliminating the Charcot bone or infected bone, and realignment and correction of the deformity, is performed via arthrodesis with internal fixation. The bone resection is critical and needs to be aggressive in removing the diseased bone and in management of obtaining definitive anatomic alignment. The aggressive bone resection is often referred to as an internal amputation. Each deformity is patient-specific and deformity-specific. It is the senior author's preference to remove any affected bone, especially bone with positive biopsies or culture.

The aggressive resection of bone is a surgical cure achieved by removing the diseased bone (Charcot and/or infected bone). It is imperative that the surgeon resects the bone in a manner that leaves only healthy, bleeding, viable bone. The resected bone reassessed with pathologic testing and cultures. The bone resection is performed with the intent of surgical excising of the pathologic bone, creating the planes to allow correction of the underlying deformity, and putting the foot and ankle back into anatomic position. New cultures and biopsies are taken from the remaining (what is suggested as healthy) most proximal and distal locations of the bone before the reduction and fixation. Any remaining voids are either backfilled with autograft and/or allograft bone. In cases of midfoot Charcot, the entire midfoot can be resected with an internal amputation and the foot functionally shortened and stabilized with internal fixation. In cases of hindfoot or ankle Charcot deformity, the same theory and principles are maintained. The fibula can be used as a graft for corticocancellous struts, as a biologic plate to aid in fixation and stability, or put through a bone mill to aid in fusion.

Some patients require reconstruction of both the hindfoot and ankle, as well as the midfoot. In these cases, reconstruction of the most proximal segment is typically performed first. Once osseous fusion is noted via radiograph and/or computed tomography (CT) scan, and the soft tissue envelope has recovered, the midfoot reconstruction is performed barring any complications.

Results of staged protocol

Recently, the authors performed a 4-year follow-up of a retrospective review of our 30 most recent patients who underwent a staged Charcot reconstruction with a multiplanar external fixator. Subjects were excluded if they had a single-stage reconstruction. Twenty-seven subjects were identified and 26 charts were available for review. Inclusion criteria included subjects who underwent a staged Charcot reconstruction, with external fixation, wound negative pressure therapy, and arthrodesis. The average age was 60 years and the average body mass index was 37. There were 13 women 13 men. All of the subjects had underlying diabetes mellitus and diabetic peripheral neuropathy.

Ten of the 27 subjects' (37%) bone biopsies were negative for osteomyelitis. The remaining 17 subjects (63%) had a bone biopsy positive for osteomyelitis. All subjects with positive cultures completed a minimum 6-week intravenous antibiotic course. Twenty-four (92%) of the 26 subjects achieved successful limb salvage. Only 2 subjects (8%) went on to below-knee (BK) amputation.

POSTOPERATIVE MANAGEMENT

Postoperative management consists of a postoperative compressive bandage and an univalve split plaster cast[32] while keeping the patient is kept nonweightbearing. Typically, the social services department is consulted in an attempt to place the patient into a rehabilitation facility or skilled nursing facility. The postoperative univalve split plaster cast is left on for 2 weeks unless otherwise indicated. At the 2-weeks postoperative visit, another compressive bandage and a BK fiberglass case are applied. The BK cast typically left on for 6 to 8 weeks based on serial radiographs. A postoperative CT scan is commonly ordered to assess the reconstruction site. Compression support hose and moisturizing agents are ordered and recommended for long-term use to assist in the postoperative edema and to help with maintaining the soft tissues. Once bony union is achieved, a CROW walker is used as the bone continues to remodel and mature. The CROW walker provides continued support as the patient begins to ambulate in anatomic alignment and the bone is remodeling. An ankle-foot orthosis (AFO) is ordered for the months or years of transition after a CROW walker, The AFO provides continued support while bony remodeling continues and until full weightbearing is permitted. Based on the outcome and the deformity, and once complete remodeling has occurred, the attempt is made to place the patient into their regular shoes, if possible, or special custom accommodative shoes based on the deformity. In cases in which a patient may not achieve a bony union but is clinically stable and maintains anatomic alignment, the patient will remain in a brace or CROW walker. The goal is to get the patient into regular shoes, if possible, because long-term compliance with the use of braces or CROW walkers is not desirable to most patients.

SUMMARY

It has been the authors' experience that staging and being patient with this challenging multifactor complex deformities has yielded the best results. We have found that staging the surgery and being patient with the timing of the stage reconstruction allows the host patient's body to react more positively, and to respond and manage the inflammatory response often experienced by the host patient relative to the infectious process and surgery. Additionally, once relief from the initial inflammatory response of the initial surgery and management of the infection are achieved, it seems the patients respond better compared with those who undergo to acute correction. The combination of an aggressive resection (internal amputation) of the diseased bone (Charcot and/or osteomyelitis) along with intravenous antibiotics provides a definitive way of curing and treating a chronic diseased bony infection with a Charcot joint.

Successful limb salvage can be achieved with proper preoperative vascular evaluation and staged correction of the deformity. We recommend noninvasive vascular testing and, if needed, a referral to a vascular surgeon before reconstruction. Initial surgery consists of a posterior muscle lengthening, bone debridement with biopsy and culture, reduction of the deformity, stabilization with an external fixator, and negative-pressure therapy to underlying open ulcerations. When appropriate, a referral to a infectious disease specialist is made. Once the wound is completely healed, and the patient is optimized, the patient undergoes the surgical definitive reconstruction surgery. The reconstructive surgery consist of aggressive bony resection (internal amputation), deformity correction via arthrodesis with internal fixation. Following reconstruction, the patients are placed in a CROW walker, transitioned to AFO, and returned to accommodative diabetic shoe gear when appropriate.

Despite modern techniques using improved methods of fixation and improved patient selection, approximately 9% of patients with Charcot deformities who undergo surgery will require a major amputation.[36]

REFERENCES

1. Varma AK. Charcot neuroarthropathy of the foot and ankle: a review. J Foot Ankle Surg 2013;52(6):740–9.
2. La Fontaine J, Shibuya N, Sampson HW, et al. Trabecular quality and cellular characteristics of normal, diabetic, and Charcot bone. J Foot Ankle Surg 2011; 50(6):648–53.
3. Wukich DK, Sadoskas D, Vaudreuil NJ, et al. Comparison of diabetic charcot patients with and without foot wounds. Foot Ankle Int 2017;38(2):140–8.
4. Ross AJ, Mendicino RW, Catanzariti AR. Role of body mass index in acute Charcot neuroarthropathy. J Foot Ankle Surg 2013;52(1):6–8.
5. Garchar D, DiDomenico LA, Klaue K. Reconstruction of Lisfranc joint dislocations secondary to Charcot neuroarthropathy using a plantar plate. J Foot Ankle Surg 2013;52(3):295–7.

6. Schneekloth BJ, Lowery NJ, Wukich DK. Charcot neuroarthropathy in patients with diabetes: an updated systematic review of surgical management. J Foot Ankle Surg 2016;55(3):586–90.

7. Charcot JM. Sur quelques arthropathies qui paraissent dépendre d'une lésion du cerveau ou de la moelle épiniere. Arch Physiol Norn Pathol 1868;1:161–78.

8. Wukich DK, Raspovic KM, Suder NC. Prevalence of peripheral arterial disease in patients with diabetic Charcot neuroarthropathy. J Foot Ankle Surg 2016;55(4):727–31.

9. Fontaine JL, Hunt NA, Curry S, et al. Fracture healing and biomarker expression in a diabetic Zucker rat model. J Am Podiatr Med Assoc 2014;104(5):428–33.

10. Melton LJ 3rd, Riggs BL, Leibson CL, et al. A bone structural basis for fracture risk in diabetes. J Clin Endocrinol Metab 2008;93(12):4804–9.

11. Schwartz AV, Sellmeyer DE, Ensrud KE, et al. Older women with diabetes have an increased risk of fracture: a prospective study. J Clin Endocrinol Metab 2001;86(1):32–8.

12. Zaidi M. Neural surveillance of skeletal homeostasis. Cell Metab 2005;1(4):219–21.

13. Murchison R, Gooday C, Dhatariya K. The development of a Charcot foot after significant weight loss in people with diabetes: three cautionary tales. J Am Podiatr Med Assoc 2014;104(5):522–5.

14. Mabilleau G, Petrova NL, Edmonds ME, et al. Increased osteoclastic activity in acute Charcot's osteoarthopathy: the role of receptor activator of nuclear factor-kappaB ligand. Diabetologia 2008;51(6):1035–40.

15. Baumhauer JF, O'Keefe RJ, Schon LC, et al. Cytokine-induced osteoclastic bone resorption in Charcot arthropathy: an immunohistochemical study. Foot Ankle Int 2006;27(10):797–800.

16. Witzke KA, Vinik AI, Grant LM, et al. Loss of RAGE defense: a cause of Charcot neuroarthropathy? Diabetes Care 2011;34(7):1617–21.

17. Rangel ÉB, Sá JR, Gomes SA, et al. Charcot neuroarthropathy after simultaneous pancreas-kidney transplant. Transplantation 2012;94(6):642–5.

18. Del Vecchio JJ, Raimondi N, Rivarola H, et al. Charcot neuroarthropathy in simultaneous kidney–pancreas transplantation: report of two cases. Diabet Foot Ankle 2013;4.

19. Caldara R, Grispigni C, La Rocca E, et al. Acute Charcot's arthropathy despite 11 years of normoglycemia after successful kidney and pancreas transplantation. Diabetes Care 2001;24(9):1690.

20. Zou RH, Wukich DK. Outcomes of foot and ankle surgery in diabetic patients who have undergone solid organ transplantation. J Foot Ankle Surg 2015;54(4):577–81.

21. Wilson M. "Charcot's neuroarthropathy after simultaneous pancreas-kidney transplant: a case report. J Am Podiatr Med Assoc 2016;106(4):294–8.

22. Smets YF, van der Pijl JW, de Fijter JW, et al. Low bone mass and high incidence of fractures after successful simultaneous pancreas-kidney transplantation. Nephrol Dial Transplant 1998;13(5):1250–5.

23. La Fontaine J, Chen C, Hunt N, et al. Type 2 diabetes and metformin influence on fracture healing in an experimental rat model. J Foot Ankle Surg 2016;55(5):955–60.

24. Pinzur MS, Lio T, Posner M. Treatment of Eichenholtz stage I Charcot foot arthropathy with a weight bearing total contact cast. Foot Ankle Int 2006;27(5):324–9.

25. Trepman E, Nihal A, Pinzur MS. Current topics review: charcot neuroarthropathy of the foot and ankle. Foot Ankle Int 2005;26(1):46–63.

26. Pinzur M. Surgical versus accommodative treatment for Charcot arthropathy of the midfoot. Foot Ankle Int 2004;25(8):545–9.
27. Snyder RJ, Frykberg RG, Rogers LC, et al. The management of diabetic foot ulcers through optimal off-loading: building consensus guidelines and practical recommendations to improve outcomes. J Am Podiatr Med Assoc 2014;104(6): 555–67.
28. González Fernández ML, Morales Lozano R, Martínez Rincón C, et al. Personalized orthoses as a good treatment option for Charcot neuro-osteoarthropathy of the foot. J Am Podiatr Med Assoc 2014;104(4):375–82.
29. Pitocco D, Ruotolo V, Caputo S, et al. Six-month treatment with alendronate in acute Charcot neuroarthropathy: a randomized controlled trial. Diabetes Care 2005;28(5):1214–5.
30. Gil J, Schiff A, Pinzur M. Cost comparison: limb salvage vs. amputation in diabetic patients with Charcot foot. Foot Ankle Int 2013;34:1097–9.
31. Pinzur MS, Evans A. Health-related quality of life in patients with Charcot foot. Am J Orthop 2003;32(10):492–6.
32. DiDomenico L, Sann P. Univalve split plaster cast for the postoperative immobilization in foot and ankle surgery. J Foot Ankle Surg 2013;52(2):260–2.
33. Williams LH, Miller DR, Fincke G, et al. Depression and incident lower limb amputations in veterans with diabetes. J Diabetes Complications 2011;25(3):175–82.
34. Jones WS, Patel MR, Dai D, et al. High mortality risks after major lower extremity amputation in Medicare patients with peripheral artery disease. Am Heart J 2013; 165(5):809–15, 815.e1.
35. DiDomenico L, Adams H, Garchar D. Endoscopic gastrocnemius recession for the treatment of gastrocnemius equinus. J Am Podiatr Med Assoc 2005;95(4): 410–3.
36. DeVries JG, Berlet G, Hyer C. A retrospective comparative analysis of Charcot ankle stabilization using an intramedullary rod with or without application of circular external fixator utilization of the retrograde arthrodesis intramedullary nail database. J Foot Ankle Surg 2012;51:420–5.
37. Lowery NJ, Woods JB, Armstrong DG, et al. Surgical management of Charcot neuroarthropathy of the foot and ankle: a systematic review. Foot Ankle Int 2012;33:113–21.
38. Crim B, Lowery N, Wukich D. Internal fixation techniques for midfoot Charcot neuroarthropathy in patients with diabetes. Clin Podiatr Med Surg 2011;28:673–85.
39. Sohn M-W, Stuck RM, Pinzur M, et al. Lower-extremity amputation risk after charcot arthropathy and diabetic foot ulcer. Diabetes Care 2010;33(1):98–100.
40. Aragón-Sánchez J, Lázaro-Martínez JL, Quintana-Marrero Y, et al. Charcot neuroarthropathy triggered and complicated by osteomyelitis. How limb salvage can be achieved. Diabet Med 2013;30(6).e229–32.

The Evolution of Limb Deformity

What Has Changed over the Past Ten Years?

Jessica L. Wilczek, DPM*, Guido A. LaPorta, DPM, MS

KEYWORDS

- Deformity • Limb • Correction • Planning • External fixation

KEY POINTS

- Evaluation of deformity on standard radiographs fosters the notion that lower extremity deformity is 2-dimensional.
- The extremity is, however, a 3-dimensional structure and deformity usually occurs in 3 planes.
- The initial step in accurate correction involves the ability to assess this 3-dimensional deformity.
- All bone deformities can be characterized by 6 parameters, 3 angulations, and 3 translations.
- The complexity of these deformities may make acute correction difficult and in some cases impossible.

INTRODUCTION

Traditional revisional, reconstructive, and deformity correction surgery of the foot, ankle, and distal tibia is usually accomplished by acute correction followed by internal fixation. Certain clinical situations, such as segmental osseous defects, osteomyelitis, Charcot foot and ankle, multiplane deformities, and soft tissue loss may be more amenable to external fixation. External fixation can be used for acute or gradual correction either by traditional Ilizarov methods or computer hexapod–assisted devices such as the Taylor spatial frame (TSF). Regardless of the strategy, the surgeon must be knowledgeable about deformity planning, osteotomy principles, and the tension-stress effect[1,2] on bone and soft tissue. This article presents the fundamental concepts necessary to successfully apply the TSF for foot and ankle deformity.

The authors have nothing to disclose.
Department of Graduate Medical Education and Podiatric Surgery, Our Lady of Lourdes Memorial Hospital, 169 Riverside Drive, Binghamton, NY 13905, USA
* Corresponding author.
E-mail address: jessicawdpmlourdes@gmail.com

TAYLOR SPATIAL FRAME

The TSF represents an elegant advancement to the Ilizarov external fixation system. Designed by J. Charles and Harold S. Taylor in 1994 and used in clinical practice since 1996, the TSF, in its basic form, is represented by 2 rings (or ring segments) connected by 6 telescopic struts with special connecting bolts. The struts are free to rotate at their connection points to the proximal and distal rings. Adjusting the length of the struts will reposition 1 ring with respect to the other. The TSF applies the concept of the Stewart[3] platform and Chasles[4] theorem to correct both 1 and 2 level deformities. The Stewart platform,[5] which serves as the basis for flight simulation, uses 6 struts and can move an object in space in any direction by adjusting the length of the struts. Correction of length, angulation, translation, or rotation, either sequentially or simultaneously, can be accomplished with the same basic construct. The number of struts coincides with the number of correction axes and provides appropriate stability to the construct. Each strut of the TSF is axially loaded without bending forces. The orientation of the struts is triangular rather than circular, resembling a very stable octahedron (crystalline structure of diamonds). The TSF has 1.1 times the axial stiffness, 2 times the bending stiffness, and 2.3 times the torsional stiffness when compared with a traditional Ilizarov-type circular frame.[6]

The TSF can be prebuilt to mimic a particular deformity (chronic method) or the rings may be individually applied, as perpendicular as possible, to its respective osseous segment with telescopic struts applied as a final step (rings first method). The authors have generally used the rings first method for most foot and ankle deformities. Specialized constructs, available since 2004, have been designed for foot deformities. The workhorse constructs for most foot deformities are the butt frame and miter frame. A lobe frame is also available but rarely used because of stability concerns.

SYSTEM COMPONENTS

The components of the TSF provide the same versatility and flexibility as the original Ilizarov system. The use of these components will not be discussed in detail here. One important feature is the presence of tabs on the rings, ring segments, and foot plates that serve as attachments for the adjustable struts. One of these tabs is designated the master tab and has a specific position and importance. During frame assembly, the following principles must be adhered to. First, the master tab is always located on the proximal ring regardless of which ring is chosen as the reference ring. When using a proximal reference, the master tab references the position of the entire construct. Therefore, second, the master tab should always be located directly anterior. If it is not directly anterior, a rotary frame offset, representing the amount of internal or external rotation of the master tab, must be entered in the software. It should be noted that most foot constructs have a 180° rotary frame offset because the master tab is located directly posterior to the leg or plantar to the foot as opposed to anterior. Third, the master tab serves as the connection for struts 1 and 2. Fourth, looking at the construct from the proximal to the distal ring, the struts are arranged from 1 through 6 in a counterclockwise direction regardless of which extremity the frame is applied to. Fifth, when using a distal reference, the tab located between struts 1 and 2 on the distal ring is used as the anterior reference. This tab is referred to as the anti–master tab and should be located directly anterior to the distal fragment. Should it not be directly anterior, a rotary frame offset representing the amount of internal or external rotation of the anti–master tab must be entered in the software.

Many foot constructs use a partial ring distally, open on the plantar side. The position directly opposite the master tab (between struts 1 and 2) is, therefore, an open space. This open space is referred to as a virtual tab and should be located directly plantar to the plane of the forefoot. This position is characterized as having a 180° rotary frame offset. Should the virtual tab not be directly plantar to the plane of the forefoot, the rotary frame offset should reflect the amount of degrees internal or external to the 180° position. The position of this virtual anti–master tab represents the orientation of the entire construct.

DEFORMITY PLANNING

A radiograph may be considered the projection of a deformity onto a reference plane (radiograph film). Therefore, using radiographs to assess deformity may be considered an exercise in projective geometry. Six deformity parameters are required to characterize any osseous deformity. Three projected angles (rotations) and 3 projected displacements (translations) can be measured on radiograph and by clinical examination.

The 3-axis rotations represent angulation in each of 2 orthogonal radiographs (anterior-posterior [AP] and lateral) and 1 clinical rotation measurement (axial rotation). The tangent of each angle, plotted perpendicular to its respective plane, describes a final rotation axis (vector sum of the 3 contributing axes) known as the Chasles axis.[4] These values are assigned positive and negative values based on the direction of rotation of each angle and the direction of displacement of each translation. The positive and negative values are determined by the mathematical convention of coordinate axes and the right-hand rule. Chasles[4] demonstrated that rotation about this single oblique axis can recreate or correct a deformity. Additionally, Chasles[4] demonstrated that displacement of this axis from the center of the fragment will provide translation in 2 planes. Progression of the fragment along this axis during rotation provides the third translation. Fortunately, the TSF can be used clinically even without knowledge of the Chasles axis.

Over the years, technology has allowed for advancements in the way radiographs are taken and used by physicians. Using a picture archiving and communication system (PACS) has become the gold standard for computer software–aided surgical planning and was found to have intraobserver and interobserver reliability similar to that of drawing and measuring off of hard copies.[7–9] A study by Khakharia and colleagues[10] compared inter-rater and intraobserver reliability to assess accuracy and reproducibility in measuring limb length discrepancies on PACS versus 51-inch hard copy radiographs. They found no difference between them, concluding that the transition to PACS for performing measurements in patients with limb length discrepancies can be made with confidence.[10]

PACS has been made easier and more user-friendly thanks to computer programs like TraumaCAD, which has assistive measures, such as illustrations or short text descriptions of anatomic landmarks in the lower limb, along with a deformity wizard tool to correctly identify the center of deformity and perform a proposed virtual osteotomy.[11] Although extremely helpful, the initial investment for programs such as this can be costly. Bone Ninja is a mobile application, available mainly for iPad usage, that allows for preplanning of deformity correction by making virtual osteotomies so that a desired outcome can be visualized. This is much less expensive than similar devices and is also conveniently located on a handheld tablet. Given that there has been an explosion in the portable medical applications market with an increase in tablet ownership of almost 30% from 2011 to 2014,[12,13] it seems appropriate that a tablet-derived application made for surgeon convenience would be desirable. Whitaker and colleagues[14,15] in a 2016 article presented in *The Journal of Children's*

Orthopedics compared PACS and Bone Ninja for assessment of lower extremity limb length discrepancy and alignment. They found no statistically significant differences in leg length discrepancy, medial proximal tibial angle (MPTA) or lateral distal femoral angle (LDFA) measurements between these 2 programs. They also found that the intraobserver and interobserver intraclass correlation coefficients for limb length, LDFA, and MPTA were also similar, thus concluding that Bone Ninja was an accurate and convenient alternative to the current gold standard of PACS in the role of deformity planning.

All 6 deformity parameters can be corrected by a circular fixator using the methods of Ilizarov,[1] which he explained through the tension-stress model in canine tibiae. Hinges, together with lengthening, translation, and rotation mechanisms, are applied either simultaneously or sequentially to correct deformity. This process, however, can be time-consuming, technically difficult, and prolong treatment programs. The TSF, assisted by computer software, provides the surgeon the ability to correct a 6-axis deformity around a single axis simultaneously or sequentially without modifying the basic construct.

CHOOSING A REFERENCE FRAGMENT AND ORIGIN

Either the proximal or distal segment can be designated as the reference fragment. Taylor[16] lists 2 criteria for the reference fragment. First, the anatomic planes of the fragment chosen should closely match the planes of the AP and lateral radiographs. Second, the AP and lateral radiographs should include the actual or anticipated level of attachment of a ring to the reference fragment. The foot (short fragment) is the best choice for the reference fragment in foot, ankle, and supramalleolar deformities; therefore, most corrections involve a distal reference.

The mechanical or anatomic axis of the reference fragment and the mechanical or anatomic axis of the moving fragment are most commonly used to determine origin and corresponding point. The intersection of these axes identifies the apex of the deformity. The axis lines create 2 transverse angles and 2 longitudinal angles centered along the center of rotation of angulation (CORA). These angles may be labeled proximal, distal, medial, and lateral angles. The proximal and distal angles are always equal and the medial and lateral angles are always equal. A line that divides an angle into 2 equal angles is called a bisector line. The transverse bisector line (tBL) bisects the medial-lateral angles. The longitudinal bisector line (lBL) bisects the proximal-distal angles. The lBL and tBL are always perpendicular to each other. The apex of the deformity establishes the location at which the tBL and lBL can be drawn. Once the bisector lines are established, any point along those lines can serve as a CORA. The axis of correction (ACA) passes through 1 of the CORAs. Movement of the ACA along the lBL produces translation without a change in length. The axes become parallel but not collinear. Movement of the ACA along the tBL produces a change in length without translation. The axes become collinear.[6] One of the CORAs is usually a good choice for the origin. The level of the apex, or CORA, should be the same on both the AP and lateral radiograph.

The origin is always located on the reference fragment and the corresponding point is always located on the moving fragment. Any point may be chosen as the origin as long as its corresponding point can be identified. In pure rotational (angulation) deformities occurring in 1 plane without any translations, the origin and corresponding point may be the same point.

Additional, or extrinsic information may influence the location of the origin. This is of particular importance when shortening is an integral part of the deformity. The amount of shortening (extrinsic information) is incorporated into both the deformity and mounting parameters. This allows correction of the entire deformity with 1 software program. Alternatively, the initial angular and translational deformity may be corrected and followed by a residual correction to address length.

SOFTWARE PARAMETERS

Deformity correction requires a thorough knowledge of deformity planning using the CORA method described by Paley.[6] This requires weightbearing, orthogonal radiographs of the extremity taken in the anatomic position. Six deformity parameters, 3 frame parameters, 4 mounting parameters, and the structure at risk (SAR) are entered into a Web-based software program. The software will generate a prescription listing daily length changes for all 6 struts and when struts need to be exchanged for an alternate size.

Deformity parameters refer to the magnitude and direction of AP view angulation, lateral view angulation, and axial angulation (clinical measurement of internal or external rotation). Single-plane angular deformities are consistent regardless of whether a proximal or distal reference is used. Varus deformities are always apex lateral, valgus deformities are always apex medial, procurvatum deformities are always apex anterior, and recurvatum deformities are always apex posterior. Internal rotations are always apex lateral and external rotations are always apex medial. High arch cavus feet are always apex dorsal and low arch flatfeet or rocker bottom feet are always apex plantar.

Additionally, AP view translation, lateral view translation, and axial translation (long or short) are entered as deformity parameters. Translation (displacement) is the perpendicular distance from the origin on the reference fragment to the corresponding point on the moving fragment. The choice of a reference fragment will affect the character of the translation. In purely translational deformities, distal reference AP view translation, and lateral view translation will generally be opposite the translation if a proximal reference is chosen. If a proximal reference describes the forefoot medially translated to the hindfoot, a distal reference will describe that same deformity as the hindfoot being laterally translated to the forefoot.

The presence of angulation in 2 planes creates the situation in which the magnitudes and directions of the 6 deformity parameters may be different depending on choice of reference fragment. Taylor[16] observed that deformity parameters viewed from 1 perspective (proximal reference) may differ from those viewed from the alternate perspective (distal reference). Although both perspectives accurately define the deformity, they are referenced to different coordinate planes. Taylor[16] referred to this phenomenon as parallactic homologues. This suggests that the clinical examination, radiographs, and frame construction should all be conducted using the same perspective. If the deformity is described relative to a proximal reference but a frame is applied relative to a distal reference perspective, the skeletal deformity may be incompletely corrected.

Mounting parameters refer to the position of the center of the reference ring to the origin (intrinsic or extrinsic). The tibia in the AP view should be centered in the ring when viewed from the front. The AP view frame offset is the distance measured from the origin to the geometric centerline of the reference ring if the tibia is shifted from center of ring. In the lateral view, the tibia is generally anterior to the geometric center of the ring. The lateral view frame offset is the distance measured from the origin to the centerline of the reference ring (the tibia is usually anterior to the geometric center of the ring). Axial frame offset is the distance measured parallel to the centerline from the origin to the center of the reference ring. These measurements are in millimeters. These mounting parameters are critical because they represent 3 intersecting planes. The point at which these planes intersect represent the virtual hinge around which correction will occur.

Rotary frame offset is the rotational position of the proximal ring relative to the proximal fragment (proximal reference) or the position of the distal ring relative to the distal fragment (distal reference). The preferred position aligns the master tab (struts 1 and 2) directly anterior to the proximal fragment or the anti–master tab (the tab located between struts 1 and 2) directly anterior to the distal fragment.

Frame parameters record the inner diameters of the proximal and distal rings or ring segments, their orientation and the 6 current strut settings.

LOCAL LENGTH ANALYSIS

The amount of shortening may be determined by geometric or trigonometric methods. The geometric method measures the perpendicular distance from the origin to the convex cortex of the reference fragment (W). Draw a line (T) the same length as W. One end of this line should rest on the plane of the origin and the opposite end should touch the mechanical axis of the deformed fragment. The point of contact of this line with the mechanical axis of the deformed fragment is the corresponding point for the chosen origin. The distance between the origin and corresponding point represents the amount of shortening.

The trigonometric method measures the distance from the origin to the convex cortex (W). Measure the angle of deformity. Shortening (S) equals $W \times \sin \Theta$. In the foot, 5 mm of shortening is arbitrarily chosen when correcting angular deformities to prevent the fragments from abutting during correction.

STRUCTURES AT RISK

SARs are generally located on the concave side of the deformity and can be defined as bone, tendon, neurovascular bundle, skin, or skin graft, which needs to be protected during correction. The peroneal nerve is generally at risk during correction of external rotation or valgus deformities. The tibial nerve is generally at risk during correction of internal rotation or varus deformities. The Achilles tendon insertion may be at risk during equinus correction. The concave side of a bone may be at risk during opening-wedge angular correction and, conversely, the convex side may be at risk during closing-wedge angular correction. The position of the SAR in reference to the origin is measured in the AP, lateral, and axial plane. This SAR measurement is the primary factor in determining the correction time. To determine the minimum correction time, the surgeon must enter a maximum safe distraction rate (MSDR). The MSDR is generally 1 mm per day for bone and may increase up to 3 mm per day for soft tissue. The SAR is the rate-limiting factor in TSF deformity correction. The surgeon may override the correction time but it is generally not recommended.

DEFORMITY PLANNING STRATEGIES

Deformity planning can be accomplished by several methods, including fracture, bisector, CORAgin, CORAsponding point, and line of closest approach. Most foot deformities use the CORAsponding point method with the possible exception of ankle equinus, which may be more amenable to the CORAgin method. The CORAsponding point method earmarks the CORA as the corresponding point. This eliminates translations from the deformity parameters.

OSTEOTOMY PRINCIPLES

There are 3 osteotomy principles that govern deformity correction. The first principle states that if the osteotomy and ACA are located on the tBL at CORA, the entire deformity will be corrected by an angulation-only osteotomy without any translation. The result is that the proximal and distal axis will be collinear.

The second principle states that if the osteotomy is performed at a distance from CORA but the ACA is located at CORA, the axis will also become collinear but will be accomplished by angulation-translation. Osteotomies may need to be performed at a distance from CORA because of anatomic considerations, diminished bone quality, previous infection, or at-risk soft tissue considerations.

The third principle states that if the osteotomy and ACA are both located at a distance from CORA, the axes will become parallel but not collinear. In effect, a deformity is corrected by creating a deformity. Osteotomy principle 3 should be avoided at all costs.

WEB-BASED SOFTWARE PROGRAM

The software program contains 7 pages that must be populated to generate a prescription for deformity correction.

Page 1 (case information): Enter case name, date, case identification, and case notes. Select a correction area from the skeleton. When choosing the foot, select which type of frame will be used (6 × 6 miter, 6 × 6 butt, or 6 + 6 ankle). Within the foot, choose a forefoot, midfoot, or hindfoot region. If ankle is chosen, there is no region to select. A preview box will display the frame chosen and the moving struts along with regions that can be corrected. Finally, choose the operating mode, either "Total Residual: or "Chronic." The total residual mode is used when the frame is applied acutely to the limb, strut lengths are entered, and the program calculates final strut lengths.

Page 2 (deformity): A proximal or distal reference must be selected. The origin is always on the reference (stationary) fragment and the corresponding point is always on the moving fragment. There are 6 required deformity parameters that characterize the deformity at the time the frame is applied. All deformities have a magnitude and direction. Not all planes will necessarily have a deformity. If there is no deformity, leave the area blank. If there is shortening or if there may be impingement, one may choose to select "Apply Axial Translation First," which prompts the software to correct shortening first. A graphic representation of the deformity is also provided.

Page 3 (frame): Select the rings and struts used for the frame. The proximal and distal ring needs to be entered. When entering a 2/3 ring, U-plate, or footplate, describe the opening from the dropdown orientation menu. The 2/3 ring and U-plates have both inner and outer mounts that must be identified. Full circles represent standard mounts and half circles represent alternate mounts. Finally, struts must be entered. There are standard and fast Fx struts, which can be entered in any combination.

Page 4 (mount): This describes the position of the center of the reference ring in relation to the origin. There are 4 required mounting parameters (AP view, lateral view, axial view, and rotary frame offset).

Page 5 (strut settings): The initial 6 strut settings are entered. The software calculates the final strut setting, which represents the settings on the final day of correction. A graphic representation of the initial and corrected frame is provided. If the chronic mode is selected, the neutral frame height and neutral strut length are entered on this page.

Page 6 (duration or SAR): The position of the SAR is described in relation to the origin in the AP, lateral and axial views. This determines the rate of correction. The SAR is indicated by a yellow circle in the graphic. Enter an MSDR. The software displays the correction time, which the surgeon may override to better control the duration of correction.

Page 7 (prescription): The prescription outlines the daily schedule of strut changes and the colored areas denote when strut changes need to be performed. It will also list the size of the struts that they need to be changed to. A new total residual program can be started on any day and one may visualize the appearance of the frame at any time during the correction. A report can be generated that lists all the pertinent information entered into the software.

The mechanical accuracy, with manual strut adjustment, for a 6-axis deformity has been measured to within 0.7° and 2 mm.

DISCUSSION

Evaluation of deformity on standard radiographs fosters the notion that lower extremity deformity is 2-dimensional. The extremity is, however, a 3-dimensional structure and deformity usually occurs in 3 planes. The initial step in accurate correction involves the ability to assess this 3-dimensional deformity. All bone deformities can be characterized by 6 parameters, 3 angulations, and 3 translations. The complexity of these deformities may make acute correction difficult and, in some cases, impossible. Additionally, factors such as soft tissue or bone infection, neurovascular considerations, and anatomy may favor gradual corrections. Gradual corrections are typically accomplished by external fixation. Circular frames using the Ilizarov[1] method offer the most comprehensive approach for deformity correction but 6-axis corrections may require frequent frame adjustments and component exchanges. Computer hexapod–assisted podiatric surgery allows gradual correction of all components of a deformity around a virtual hinge. The TSF provides the surgeon with a stable and accurate method for managing complex deformity about the foot, ankle, and lower leg. Changes or alterations to the correction plan are computer-driven, obviating return to the operating room.

The TSF has been used successfully over the past 15 years to treat deformities of the foot and ankle[17–21] and has gained wide acceptance in orthopedic trauma. In a recent review from 2016, the fixator had produced excellent results in the management of complex tibial nonunions with a 95% mean patient satisfaction score.[22] The dynamic hexapod system has been studied in the literature with respect to its functionality compared with its predecessor, the standard Ilizarov-style uniplanar external fixation device. In a study aimed at determining the differences between them when biomechanical normal gait was encountered (eg, axial compressing, bending, and rotation torque), the TSF was found to be less rigid than the Ilizarov frame under axial load but more rigid under bending and torsional load. However, the axial rigidity and, therefore, stiffness increased in the TSF with the use of half pins, which was then comparable with the wire system in an Ilizarov external device. The investigators concluded that the TSF, when half pins are used, is a more resistant construct to normal physiologic biomechanical stress than the traditional Ilizarov device.[23] Reitenbach and colleagues[24] compared limb lengthening and minimal deformity correction using Ilizarov external fixation or TSF in a total of 43 subjects. They found statistically significant differences in axial deviation at follow-up (TSF 0%, Ilizarov frame 36.8%), as well as statistically significantly fewer complications according to the Paley[6] criteria in the TSF group versus the Ilizarov[1] group, as well as a drastically lower number of pin tract infections in the TSF group (TSF 12.1%, Ilizarov 50%, and TSF 9.1%, Ilizarov

40%, respectively). A comparison of cost and complications between uniplanar versus TSF external fixation for pediatric diaphyseal tibial fractures was conducted by Shore and colleagues[25] in 2016. The findings included a statistically significant earlier time to union in the TSF group and statistically significantly fewer postoperative complications, mainly pin tract infections. Although initial cost of the fixators was quite different ($5074.00 for the uniplanar device vs $10,675 for the TSF), corrected cost analysis to account for return operating room charges secondary to postoperative complications lead to no difference between the 2 devices in overall cost of treatment.

Significantly, although TSF was the first marketed hexapod frame for the intended purposes of limb deformity correction, there have been other systems developed that are considered comparable. The MAXFRAME was introduced by DePuy Synthes (Synthes USA, LLC, Monument, CO). It, too, is a multiaxial correction system with computer-assisted correction capabilities. Indications for this frame include open and closed fractures, pseudoarthrosis, limb lengthening, arthrodesis, nonunions, correction of bony or soft tissue deformities, and the correction of segmental defects. It is intended for use in the pediatric and adult populations. The design includes full circular rings, 5/8 rings, and foot plates. It also includes standard struts and quick adjust struts, the latter providing an audible click with every 1 mm of rotation. As with other systems, mounting parameters must be established, noting the amount of offset between the frame and the proximal reference point. Alternatively, one can establish a distal reference, as with a distal tibial fracture, and the computer should generate a prescription for correction easily in either scenario. Orthofix Orthopedic Company (Lewisville, TX) introduced its version of the hexapod frame, TL-HEX, which has many components compatible with their static frame, the True-Lok, creating interchangeable systems with the ability to gradually correct multiplane deformities. This system has its own computer-generated prescription and associated software. Stryker Orthopedics (Stryker Corporation, Kalamazoo, MI) has also developed their dynamic hexapod frame, which includes a technologically advanced strut adjustment system that requires no daily turns by the patient but instead relies on radiofrequency communication through a simple handheld device.

The major obstacle to successful use of the TSF or any dynamic hexapod frame is a steep learning curve. The surgeon must be knowledgeable about deformity principles, osteotomy rules, structures at risk, and anatomic safe zones, in addition to being familiar with the application of external fixation. Once mastered, no more powerful tool exists for the correction of musculoskeletal deformity.

REFERENCES

1. Ilizarov GA. The tension-stress effect on the genesis and growth of tissues: Part II. The influence of the rate and frequency of distraction. Clin Orthop Relat Res 1989;(239):249–81, 263–85.
2. Bauchau O, Trainelli L. The vectorial parameterization of rotation. Nonlinear Dyn 2003;32(1):71–92.
3. Stewart DA. Platform with six degrees of freedom. Proc Inst Mech Eng 1965; 180(15):371–86.
4. Chasles M. Note sur les proprieties generals du systeme de deux corps semblables entr'eux. Bulletin des Sciences Mathematiques, Astronomiques, Physiques et Chemiques 1830;14:321–6 [in French].
5. Beggs JS. Advanced mechanism. New York: Macmillan Company; 1966.
6. Paley D. Principles of deformity correction. Berlin, Germany: Springer-Verlag Berlin Heidelberg; 2002. p. 61–189.

7. Sabharwal S, Zhao C, McKeon J, et al. Reliability analysis for radiographic measurement of limb length discrepancy: full-length standing anteroposterior radiograph versus scanogram. J Pediatr Orthop 2007;27(1):46–50.

8. Marx RG, Grimm P, Lillemoe KA, et al. Reliability of lower extremity alignment measurement using radiographs and PACS. Knee Surg Sports Traumatol Arthrosc 2011;19(10):1693–8.

9. Hankemeier S, Gosling T, Richter M, et al. Computer-assisted analysis of lower limb geometry: higher intraobserver reliability compared to conventional method. Comput Aided Surg 2006;11(2):81–6.

10. Khakharia S, Bigman D, Fragomen AT, et al. Comparison of PACS and hardcopy 51-inch radiographs for measuring leg length and deformity. Clin Orthop Relat Res 2011;469(1):244–50.

11. Steinberg EL, Segev E, Drexler M, et al. Preoperative planning of orthopedic procedures using digitalized software systems. Isr Med Assoc J 2016;18(6):354–8.

12. Franko OI. Smartphone apps for orthopedic surgeons. Clin Orthop Relat Res 2011;469(7):2042–8.

13. Mosa AS, Yoo I, Sheets L. A systematic review of healthcare applications for smartphones. BMC Med Inform Decis Mak 2012;12:67.

14. Whitaker AT, Gesheff MG, Jauregui JJ, et al. Comparison of PACS and Bone Ninja mobile application for assessment of lower extremity limb length discrepancy and alignment. J Child Orhop 2016;10:439–43.

15. Gessmann J, Jettkant B, Königshausen M, et al. Improved wire stiffness with modified connection bolts in Ilizarov external frames: a biomechanical study. Acta Bioeng Biomech 2012;14(4):15–21.

16. Taylor JC. Six-axis deformity analysis and correction. In: Paley D, editor. Principles of deformity correction. Berlin/Heidelberg/New York: Springer; 2002. p. 411–36.

17. Eidelman M, Bialik V, Katzman A. Correction of deformities in children using the Taylor spatial frame. J Pediatr Orthop B 2006;15:387–95.

18. Eidelman M, Katzman A. Treatment of complex foot deformities in children with the Taylor spatial frame. Orthopedics 2008;31(10).

19. Fadel M, Hosny G. The Taylor spatial frame for deformity correction in the lower limbs. Int Orthop 2005;29:125–9.

20. Feldman DS, Shin SS, Madan S, et al. Correction of tibial malunion and nonunion with six-axis analysis deformity correction using the Taylor Spatial Frame. J Orthop Trauma 2003;17(8):549–54.

21. Waizy H, Windhagen H, Stukenborg-Colsman C, et al. Taylor spatial frame in severe foot deformities using double osteotomy: technical approach and primary results. Int Orthop 2011;35(10):1489–95.

22. Khunda A, Al-Maiyah M, Eardley WGP, et al. The management of tibial fracture non-union using the Taylor Spatial Frame. J Orthop 2016;13(4):360–3.

23. Henderson DJ, Rushbrook JL, Harwood PJ, et al. What are the biomechanical properties of the Taylor spatial frame? Clin Orthop Relat Res 2017;475(5):1472–82.

24. Reitenbach E, Rodl R, Gosheger G, et al. Deformity correction and extremity lengthening in the lower leg: comparison of clinical outcomes with two external surgical procedures. Springerplus 2016;5(1):2003.

25. Shore BJ, DiMauro JP, Spence DD, et al. Uniplanar versus Taylor spatial frame external fixation for pediatric diaphyseal tibia fractures: a comparison of cost and complications. J Pediatr Orthop 2016;36(8):821–8.

The Role of Polyvinyl Alcohol in Cartilage Repair of the Ankle and First Metatarsophalangeal Joint

Thomas J. Chang, DPM

KEYWORDS

- Cartiva implant • Polyvinyl alcohol • First metatarsophalangeal joint

KEY POINTS

- The Cartiva implant (Cartiva, Alpharetta, GA) is an exciting option in dramatically diminishing patient symptoms in advanced stages of hallux rigidus as well as allowing continued joint motion.
- The procedure does not burn many bridges in case a future revision to an arthrodesis is necessary.
- This advantage is in contradistinction to other current implants whereby more bone resection is required for implant placement.

Since July 2016, there has been an exciting new option in treating patients with hallux rigidus in a foot and ankle practice. Clearly, cheilectomy and first metatarsophalangeal joint (MPJ) fusions have been the standard approach for hallux rigidus. In addition to these two orthopedic standards, osteotomies and implants (both hemi and total option) have been popularized within the literature. There have also been a variety of first MPJ hemi and total implants, which are also discussed. Although all of these have been reported in literature, there is still a concern with the long-term success of first MPJ implants in general. The more predictable option seems to be a fusion of this joint, but there are clearly patients who desire and choose to maintain their motion. We understand first MPJ fusions to be fully functional with good long-term outcomes, yet patients are limited to a 1-in heel in their shoe wear.

Although used for years in Europe and Canada, the Cartiva implant (Cartiva, Alpharetta, GA) was recently approved by the Food and Drug Administration (FDA) for use in the United States last July.

The author has nothing to disclose.
Redwood Orthopedic Surgery Associates, Inc, 208 Concourse Boulevard, #1, Santa Rosa, CA 95403, USA
E-mail address: thomaschang14@comcast.net

Clin Podiatr Med Surg 35 (2018) 133–143
https://doi.org/10.1016/j.cpm.2017.08.014
0891-8422/18/© 2017 Elsevier Inc. All rights reserved.

podiatric.theclinics.com

The material is polyvinyl alcohol and is classified as a hydrogel. There is no silicone within this device, so concerns of silicone inflammatory changes are not present. This material is used in contact lenses and has undergone extensive cyclical testing studies. The studies have loaded the implant under rotational dorsiflexion and plantar flexion movements with greater than 5 million cycles without showing any dramatic wear on the implant.

The Cartiva implant is an exciting option in dramatically diminishing patient symptoms in advanced stages of hallux rigidus as well as allowing continued joint motion. It is a procedure that also does not burn many bridges in case a future revision to an arthrodesis is necessary. This advantage is in contradistinction to other current implants whereby more bone resection is required for implant placement (**Fig 1**).

There are currently 2 published prospective studies that report on short and intermediate outcomes with this implant. In the Motion Study, authored by Baumhauer and colleagues,[1,2] this was conducted at 12 sites within the United Kingdom and Canada. Patients were randomized into either a first MPJ fusion group or a Cartiva group. A total of 236 patients were initially enrolled. The patients were surgically treated in Canada and England and have been followed up for 2 and 5 years, respectively. The functional outcome scores and visual analog scale (VAS) parameters and pain scales were all comparable, as a joint fusion and the Cartiva implant were used in a side-to-side comparison. This study was pivotal in the FDA approval in the early months of 2016. At the 5-year follow-up on this same patient pool, 29 patients were included in this article. Pain VAS and functional outcome scores continued to improve clinically to statistically significant levels. Radiographically, there were no findings of movement or implant wear or subsidence. One implant was removed and converted successfully to a fusion 2 years after surgery.

The implant is part of the cheilectomy procedure. There is a standard dorsomedial incision on the first MPJ. Dissection is carried down to the joint capsule, and then the first MPJ is exposed. A dorsal, medial, and lateral resection of bone spurs is carried out on the metatarsal head. The base of the phalanx is also inspected, and any

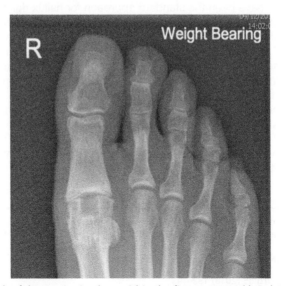

Fig. 1. Radiograph of the Cartiva in place within the first metatarsal head. There is no loss of metatarsal length.

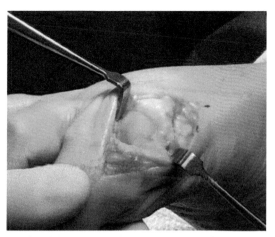

Fig. 2. Standard case of hallux rigidus with central cartilage loss and hypertrophic bone in the periphery.

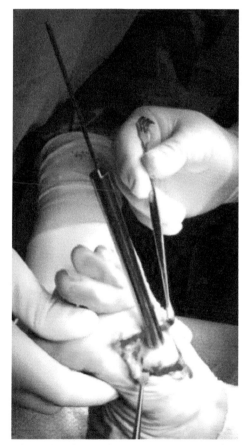

Fig. 3. Sizer for the implant placed over the central cartilage defect. Note the cannulated drill pin. The 2 sizes are 8 mm or 10 mm.

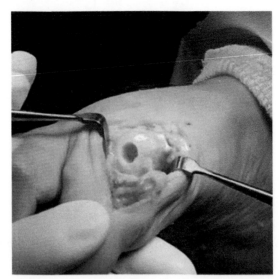

Fig. 4. Defect noted within the metatarsal head after drilling is completed. This is also drilled to a specific depth, which will allow the implant to sit proud.

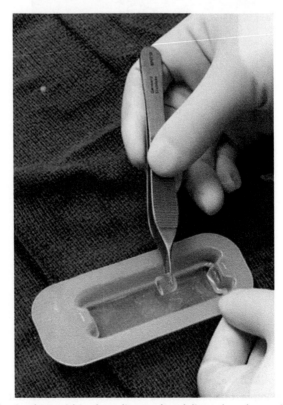

Fig. 5. The Cartiva implant within the saline packet delivered to the sterile field.

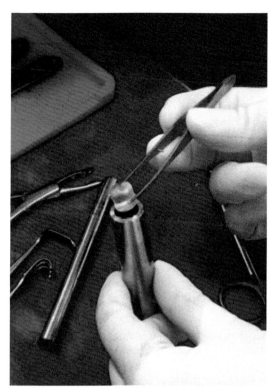

Fig. 6. The implant placed within the delivery tube.

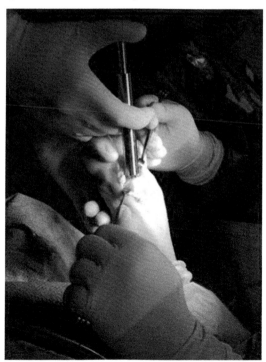

Fig. 7. The implant being placed into the metatarsal head drill hole with the use of a plunger system.

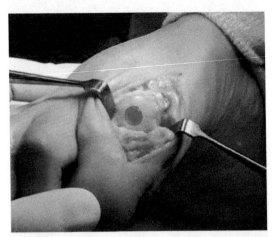

Fig. 8. Intraoperative picture of implant in place within the metatarsal head.

hypertrophic bone is cleaned off with a rongeur. The cartilage is carefully inspected, and many times an osteochondral injury will be present (**Fig 2**).

After the cheilectomy, the use of the Cartiva is considered to provide distraction or separation of the proximal phalanx from the first metatarsal head. In cases of joint narrowing and bone contact, the goal is to push the proximal phalanx away from contact

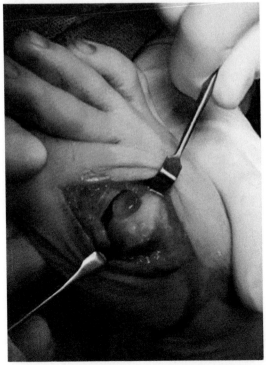

Fig. 9. Dorsal view of the implant extending off the metatarsal head a few millimeters.

with the first metatarsal head. This interpositional space acts much like a bumper, not allowing the phalangeal base to contact the metatarsal head. With this goal in mind, it is important to leave the implant proud with in the metatarsal head so it can effectively provide a buffer between the two bones. There are currently 2 sizes used in the United States, the 8-mm and the 10-mm implants (**Fig 3**). Your decision on which size to use can be determined by the size of the metatarsal head. It is usually recommended to leave a bit more of the shape of the metatarsal head when considering a Cartiva implant, rather than a resection of the dorsal third of the metatarsal head in a standard cheilectomy.

The implant is generally placed centrally within the metatarsal head but can also be directed slightly medial or lateral from the midline depending on where the osteochondral injury primarily sits and where the phalangeal contact generally occurs. The guide pin is placed within the metatarsal head, and then the appropriate sizer can be placed over this pin to look at the amount of bone that will be left supporting the implant. The next step is the most important, that is, drilling out the cylinder within the metatarsal head. This step can be aggressive, so there should be a gentle pressure on the bone as the drill contacts the metatarsal (**Fig 4**). Beware of pushing too aggressively, as the drill will bottom out quickly with mild to moderate pressure. More surgeons are now drilling to a shallower depth so the final position of the Cartiva implant will sit even

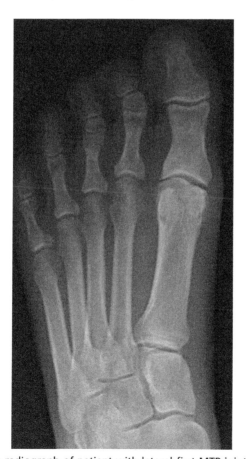

Fig. 10. Preoperative radiograph of patient with lateral first MTP joint narrowing.

prouder inside the joint (**Figs. 5–7**). With the traditional technique, the implant usually sits around 1 to 2 mm proud off the surface of the metatarsal head. In personal communication and anecdotal comments received, the preferred placement of the implant suggests that 2 to 3 mm may even be more ideal; in some cases, even 3 to 4 mm have been used. There can even be an instrument placed at the level of the metatarsal head, which acts as an earlier contact for the stop ledge on the drill, resulting in an additional millimeter or two of extra implant sitting proud within the joint. Depending on your specific goals with this implant in your patients, you may choose to have the implant sit between 2 and 4 mm proud (**Figs. 8 and 9**). There has been no evidence to show that a prouder implant has caused any negative outcomes, and it may even suggest the opposite.

Proper technique is now used to place the 8- or 10-mm implant into the metatarsal head and have the implant sit proud within the joint. With joint preservation, it is important to evaluate the sesamoids and their ability to glide underneath the metatarsal head. If any adhesions are visualized or recognized during the surgery, they should be released with a McGlamry elevator or sharp dissection. Sesamoid removal may also be indicated in specific cases. Sesamoid pathology is often the culprit in continued pain after implant and also joint preservation procedures in hallux rigidus,

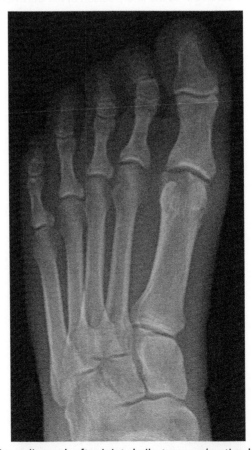

Fig. 11. Postoperative radiograph after joint cheilectomy and noticeable separation of the lateral first MTPJ joint space.

and a preoperative computed tomography scan may prove extremely useful to evaluate this sesamoid-metatarsal head articulation in decision-making.

The joint is taken through a range of motion to make sure there is freedom of movement without crepitation. The joint capsule is now closed along with the skin and a soft dressing applied. Postoperatively, patients are allowed to bear weight on their heel immediately and can also transition to putting weight through the forefoot as tolerated. Sutures remain in for roughly 2 weeks, and range of motion is encouraged from day 1.

In cases of hallux valgus with intraarticular defects, deformity correction is strongly recommended as well during implant placement. Intermetatarsal angles should be corrected, either through proximal or distal approaches as well as sagittal plane malalignment. Structural deformities within the proximal phalanx should also be addressed when necessary so the implant will sit within the best, most stable congruous joint environment after placement (**Figs. 10–15**).

There are future areas of possible indication for the location of the implant. These areas include second and lesser MPJ pathology, such as Freiberg or joint arthritis. One can also imagine this possibly being studied within the ankle joint, the talonavicular joint, and possibly as a spacer in the lateral Lisfranc region. Besides these

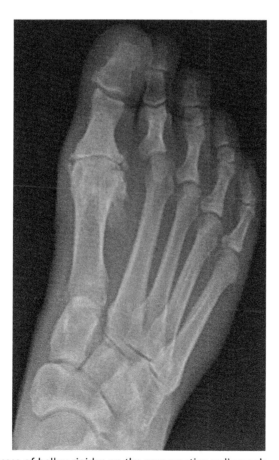

Fig. 12. Another case of hallux rigidus on the preoperative radiograph.

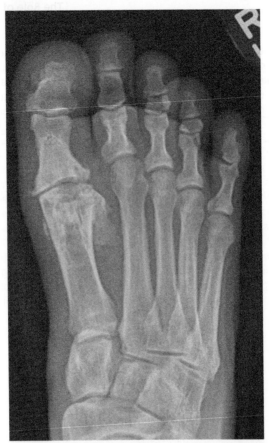

Fig. 13. Postoperative radiograph with cheilectomy and placement of the Cartiva implant.

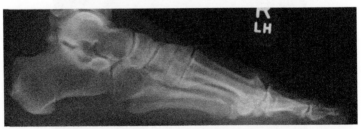

Fig. 14. Lateral preoperative radiograph with dorsal spurring from both sides of the joint.

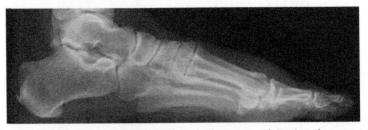

Fig. 15. Lateral postoperative radiograph after cheilectomy and Cartiva placement. There is a subtle separation of the joint space noted.

indications within the foot and ankle, there will unquestionably be uses within the hand and possibly other joints throughout the body. This new device offers an exciting option for foot and ankle surgeons as we continue to find good options for patients with debilitating hallux limitus and rigidus.

REFERENCES

1. Baumhauer JF, Singh D, Glazebrook M, et al. Prospective, randomized, multi-centered clinical trial assessing safety and efficacy of a synthetic cartilage implant versus first metatarsophalangeal arthrodesis in advanced hallux rigidus. Foot Ankle Int 2016;37(5):457–69.
2. Daniels TR, Younger AS, Penner MJ, et al. Midterm outcomes of polyvinyl alcohol hydrogel hemiarthroplasty of the first metatarsophalangeal joint in advanced hallux rigidus. Foot Ankle Int 2017;38(3):243–7.

Printed and bound by CPI Group (UK) Ltd, Croydon, CR0 4YY

07/10/2024

01040501-0013